The Art and Science of Abdominal Hernia

Edited by Muhammad Shamim

Published in London, United Kingdom

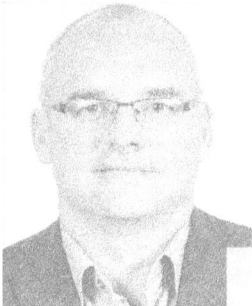
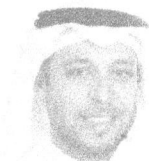
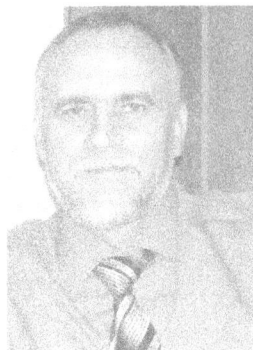
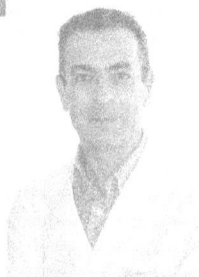
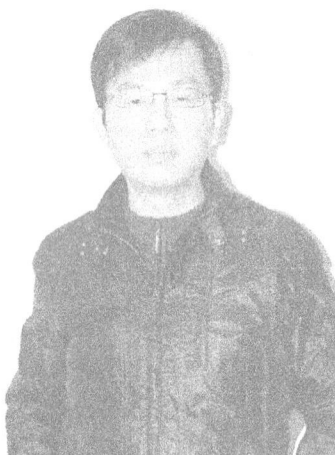
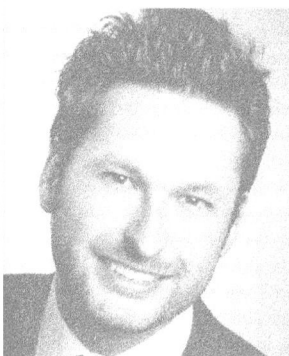
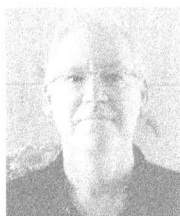

IntechOpen

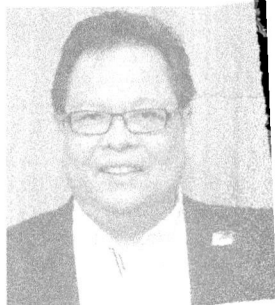
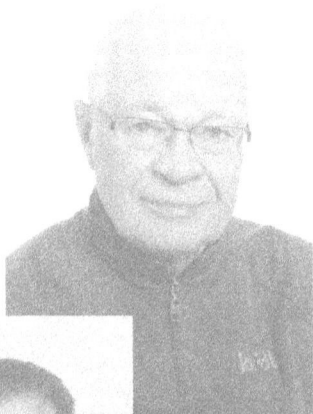
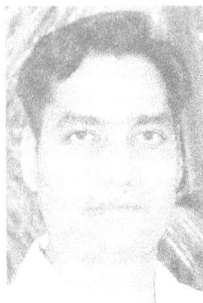
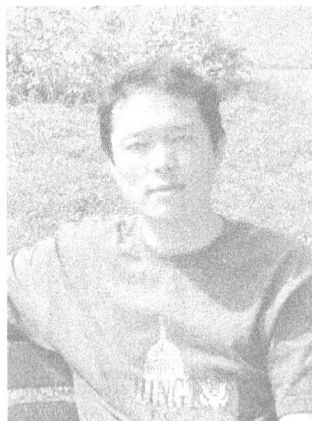
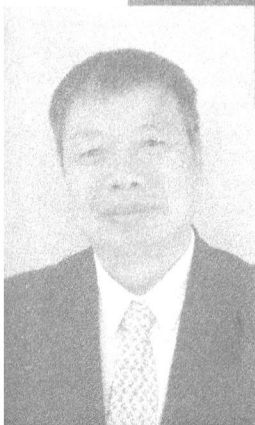
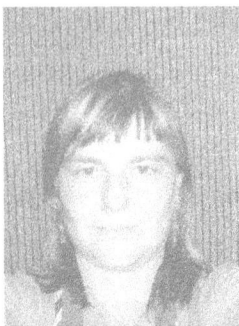

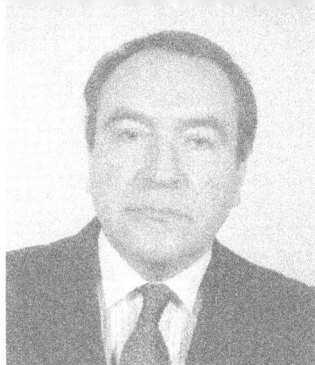

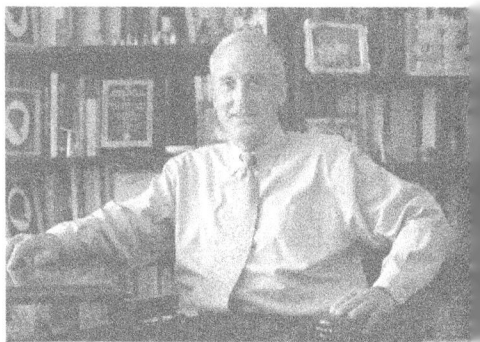

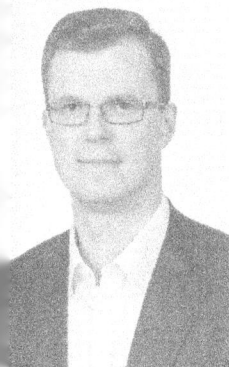

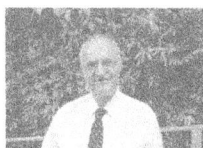

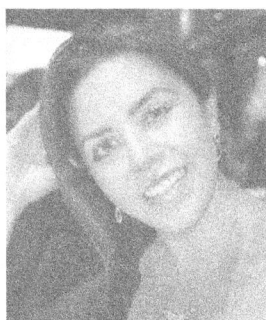

Supporting open minds since 2005

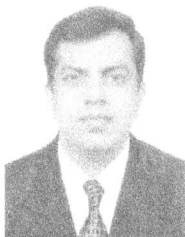

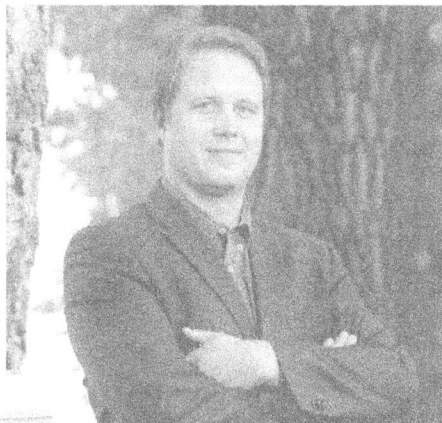

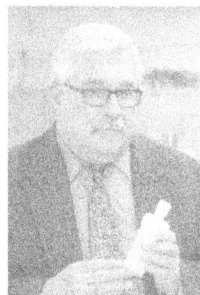

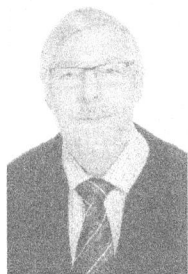

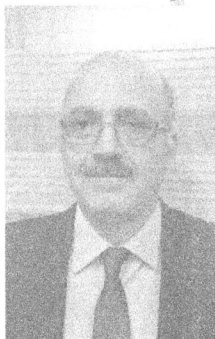

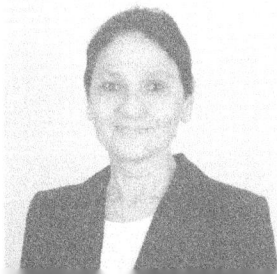

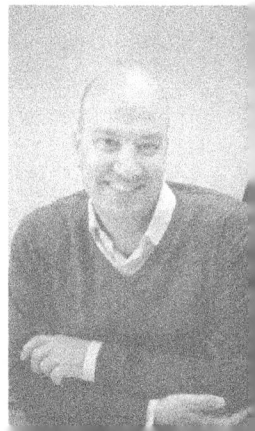

The Art and Science of Abdominal Hernia
http://dx.doi.org/10.5772/intechopen.92420
Edited by Muhammad Shamim

Contributors
Roberto Sanisidro Torre, Ibrahima Konaté, Abdourahmane Ndong, Jacques N. Tendeng, César Felipe
Ploneda-Valencia, Carlos Alfredo Bautista-López, Carlos Alberto Navarro-Montes, Juan Carlos
Verdugo-Tapia, Muhammad Shamim

Notice
Statements and opinions expressed in the chapters are these of the individual contributors and not
necessarily those of the editors or publisher. No responsibility is accepted for the accuracy of
information contained in the published chapters. The publisher assumes no responsibility for any
damage or injury to persons or property arising out of the use of any materials, instructions, methods
or ideas contained in the book.

First published in London, United Kingdom, 2022 by IntechOpen
IntechOpen is the global imprint of INTECHOPEN LIMITED, registered in England and Wales,
registration number: 11086078, 5 Princes Gate Court, London, SW7 2QJ, United Kingdom
Printed in Croatia

British Library Cataloguing-in-Publication Data
A catalogue record for this book is available from the British Library

Additional hard and PDF copies can be obtained from orders@intechopen.com

The Art and Science of Abdominal Hernia
Edited by Muhammad Shamim
p. cm.
Print ISBN 978-1-83968-332-9
Online ISBN 978-1-83968-333-6
eBook (PDF) ISBN 978-1-83968-334-3

We are IntechOpen,
the world's leading publisher of
Open Access books
Built by scientists, for scientists

5,600+
Open access books available

138,000+
International authors and editors

175M+
Downloads

Our authors are among the

156
Countries delivered to

Top 1%
most cited scientists

12.2%
Contributors from top 500 universities

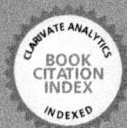

CLARIVATE ANALYTICS
BOOK
CITATION
INDEX
INDEXED

WEB OF SCIENCE™

Selection of our books indexed in the Book Citation Index (BKCI)
in Web of Science Core Collection™

Interested in publishing with us?
Contact book.department@intechopen.com

Numbers displayed above are based on latest data collected.
For more information visit www.intechopen.com

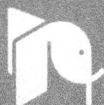

Meet the editor

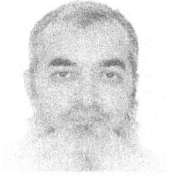

Dr. Muhammad Shamim is Assistant Professor of Surgery at College of Medicine, Prince Sattam Bin Abdulaziz University, Saudi Arabia, and Supervisor of General Surgery training at College of Physicians and Surgeons, Pakistan. He was awarded fellowships in surgery from Pakistan, the United Kingdom, and the United States, as well as master's degrees in Health Professionals Education from Netherland and Egypt. He is also the author of *Essential of Surgery, 8th edition* and *Clinical Techniques in Surgery, 2nd edition*. He has also authored several research publications and is currently a peer reviewer and editorial board member for several indexed surgery journals.

Contents

Preface

Abdominal wall hernia surgery is one of the most performed general surgical operations in the world and is considered the "bread and butter" of general surgical practice. The spectrum of surgeries includes both elective and emergency cases of different anatomical types of abdominal wall hernias, the most common being inguinal hernia. Hernia surgery has undergone a remarkable transformation during the last two decades. Advances in mesh technology as well as surgical innovations such as minimal access surgery have decreased recurrence of hernias and allowed for faster patient recuperation. Repair material has evolved from absorbable sutures to monofilament sutures to mesh and plugs. Innovations in surgical techniques developed from open herniorrhaphy techniques such as Lytle's method, Shouldice's method, Bassini's repair, and Darning's repair to open hernioplasty (Lichtenstein's repair), and finally minimal surgery approaches of laparoscopic and robotic hernia surgery. Anatomically, every hernia patient is considered different with variations in dissections. Variations in the anatomy of that hernial sac, like that of congenital inguinal hernia, require a different surgical approach during sac dissections. Similarly, variations such as a complication or an unusual content may warrant modifications in surgical techniques.

This book is a comprehensive guide to the diagnosis and management of abdominal wall hernias. It is designed to serve the broader surgical community from postgraduate students to practicing surgeons. A chapter on clinical evaluation and diagnosis highlights the importance of accurate and timely diagnosis in the management of hernia. Separate chapters are dedicated to inguinal, femoral, and umbilical hernias, which are among the most common abdominal hernias. Finally, a chapter on biological mechanisms of inguinal pain and chronification highlights the importance of continued management of hernia patients postoperatively. All chapters are written by senior experts in the field of surgery and include up-to-date scientific material.

This book would not have been possible without the extended help and support from the editorial and managing staff of IntechOpen. I am especially grateful to Author Service Manager Ms. Jasna Bozic.

Muhammad Shamim
Department of Surgery,
College of Medicine,
Prince Sattam Bin Abdulaziz University,
Alkharj, Saudi Arabia

Chapter 1

Clinical Evaluation of Abdominal Wall Hernias

Muhammad Shamim

Abstract

Hernia is defined as protrusion of a viscus or part of a viscus through a weakening or defect in the wall of its containing cavity. Areas of potential anatomical weakness includes inguinal canal, femoral canal, linea alba, umbilical scar, as well as acquired surgical trauma. The weakening/defect may be acquired (like surgical scar) or congenital (like deep inguinal ring). Raised intraabdominal pressure is the most important factor that leads to the development of hernia through the weak areas. Clinically, the hernia usually presents with an abdominal swelling that progresses gradually over time. The sites of hernia are characteristic and usually points towards the diagnosis. While evaluating a hernia clinically, it is important to identify the content of the hernia sac and whether it suffers any complication, as well as the cause of the hernia development. Failing to identify these prior to surgery, will likely result in morbidity as well as recurrence. This chapter will focus on the clinical art of history taking and examination of different abdominal hernias.

Keywords: Hernia, abdominal, clinical evaluation

1. Introduction

The abdominal wall hernia is a protrusion of an abdominal viscus or a part of a viscus through a weakness or defect in the wall. The defect may be congenital like deep inguinal ring and umbilical scar or acquired like incisional scar. The most important factor contributing to the development of hernia is the high intraabdominal pressure, first stretching the weakened area and ultimately giving way to the hernia sac. High intraabdominal pressure may result from chronic cough, straining at micturition or defecation, heavy weight lifting, pregnancy and intraabdominal malignancy. Smoking has a dual role in hernia development, contributing to chronic cough from bronchitis and muscular weakness from acquired collagen deficiency.

The clinical diagnosis of abdominal hernia is usually clear. It may be reducible and uncomplicated or irreducible with complication like obstruction, strangulation or inflammation. However, during clinical evaluation, it is important to identify the cause of hernia development, so as to address this, otherwise recurrence will be likely. It is also important to identify the content of hernia sac, as patient may develop a complication of it. The most common contents are omentum and small bowel; however, large bowel, appendix, Meckel's diverticulum, ovary, fallopian tube and urinary bladder can also occupy hernia sac, or form part of the sac as in sliding hernia.

The common varieties of abdominal herniae are inguinal, femoral, umbilical, epigastric and incisional, while obturator, lumbar, gluteal and Spigelian hernias [1] are rarer. Inguinal hernia has two varieties, direct and indirect. Direct inguinal hernia comes out through the medial half of weak posterior inguinal canal wall and then becomes superficial through superficial inguinal ring. Indirect (oblique) inguinal hernia comes out through the deep inguinal ring, traverses the inguinal canal and becomes superficial through the same superficial inguinal ring. It can occur as congenial inguinal hernia due to persistence of processus vaginalis; though congenital, it is not necessarily present at birth and may appear first time in adult life with hernia reaching to the bottom of scrotum at first appearance. Inguinal hernia is referred to as complete, when it reaches the bottom of the scrotum. The femoral hernia comes out through the femoral ring, traverses the femoral canal and becomes superficial through the saphenous opening. The umbilical hernia in infants is through the weak umbilical scar, whereas in adults it is through the linea alba just above (supraumbilical) or just below (infraumbilical) the umbilicus. The epigastric hernia occurs through the linea alba anywhere between xiphoid process and umbilicus, usually midway between these structures.

2. History taking in abdominal hernia

About 75% of all abdominal wall hernias occur in the groin area [2]. There are some age and sex characteristics. Indirect inguinal hernia usually develops in young adults, whereas direct inguinal hernia and umbilical hernia in middle aged and older patients. Inguinal hernias are more common in males (9:1 male predominance) [3] whereas femoral hernias are more common in females (4:1 female predominance) [4].

The lump is the most common complaint, with the patient noticing a swelling in one or more of the anatomical locations of hernia. It may start spontaneously as in congenital hernia or follow some abdominal straining activity as in acquired hernia. The anatomical site of first appearance is important, i.e. umbilicus, inguinal canal or femoral canal (below the groin crease). An inguinal hernia may reaches the bottom of scrotum on its first appearance, indicating a congenital hernia developing into a preformed sac. However, the usually history is of a small swelling appearing, which gradually increases in size over time (acquired hernia). A hernia may or may not reduce on lying down; direct inguinal hernia reduces automatically as soon as the patient lies down, whereas indirect inguinal, umbilical and incisional hernias either reduces slowly itself or has to be reduced manually. Femoral hernia usually can't be completely reduced.

The pain is the second important complaint. It tends to occur at some specific points in the hernia history. First, it occur in the very beginning when there is tendency to hernia, when the patient complains of a dragging and aching type of pain which gets worse as the day progresses; this pain is due to stretching of the hernia ring and it ceases once the ring become fully dilated so as to pass the sac [5]. Pain may worsen by activities that increases intraabdominal pressure like coughing, laughing, lifting or straining, as more of the abdominal content are pushing through the defect [5]. Later, the pain occur when hernia content develop some complication like strangulation, obstruction or inflammation. Groin pain, without any obvious bulge, can also occur in young athletes due to overuse injury associated with adductor muscles and tendons [6, 7]. This is vague unilateral or bilateral groin pain, usually occur on exertion and may radiates to the scrotum and medial thigh [7]. This represents sports hernia, a misnomer, not a true hernia, with a weakness of the posterior wall of the inguinal canal [7].

Finally, the patients may have some symptoms indicating the cause of hernia or a complication. So, the patients may have persistent cough of chronic bronchitis, chronic constipation or prostatism of benign prostatic hyperplasia. Similarly, patients may have cardinal symptoms of intestinal obstruction, i.e. colicky abdominal pain, abdominal distension, vomiting and absolute constipation. The past history may uncover an abdominal operation like appendicectomy, cholecystectomy or renal surgery.

3. Objective examination of abdominal hernia

The diagnosis of abdominal wall hernia can be made with reasonable accuracy through history and clinical examination. However, imaging modalities like CT scan, ultrasound and MRI can help in difficult or complicated cases. One study reported 75% sensitivity and 96% specificity of clinical examination in hernia diagnosis [8].

3.1 Positioning and exposure

The exposure must include the whole abdomen (and not limiting to just the site of complaint) from the level of xiphisternum to the mid-thigh. This is necessary to avoid missing another hernia, which the patient is not aware of. Remember, the causative factor raised intraabdominal pressure is equally applied to all anatomically weak areas.

The patient should first examine in standing position and the doctor sit in front of him/her, especially if the presenting complaint is suggesting the possibility of hernia. But, if an incidental hernia discovered during abdominal examination, then ask to stand up later. In the end, the patient is examined in lying down position for reducibility and confirming anatomical types.

3.2 Inspection

A swelling may be present or appear when the patient coughs. Note its site, size, shape, extent, impulse on cough and whether any other swelling present in scrotum or elsewhere. The site is characteristic of any abdominal wall hernia. Inguinal hernia lies above the groin crease medially, whereas femoral hernia lies below the groin crease medially. Epigastric hernia lies in the upper part of linea alba, whereas paraumbilical hernia lies in the linea alba adjacent to umbilicus. Indirect inguinal hernia is typically pyriform-shaped with its stalk at superficial inguinal ring, and extends towards and into the scrotum. Direct inguinal hernia is hemi-spherical shaped and usually don't enter into scrotum. Femoral hernia is ovoid or hemi-spherical shaped, starting below the groin crease and ascends upwards.

The presence of expansile cough impulse is diagnostic of hernia. However, it may be absent in cases of complication like obstruction/strangulation, when neck of the sac is blocked by adhesions, preventing additional viscera to enter hernial sac on coughing. Conclude the inspection by examining the skin overlying hernia and skin of penis and scrotum. Any redness is an indication of complication like inflammation and strangulation.

3.3 Percussion and auscultation

These are useful to confirm the characteristics of hernial content. The percussion will give a resonant note if the hernia contains bowel (enterocele), and a dull note if it contains omentum (omentocele). Similarly, auscultation will confirm the presence of gut if bowel sounds are there. Additionally, tenderness can be revealed on percussion, if the content is inflamed or in cases of strangulation.

3.4 Palpation

This includes palpation of the swelling, as well as scrotum and its contents (especially if the swelling is entering scrotum) and the penis and urethra. Begin with confirming the inspection findings of expansile cough impulse, as well as confirm the anatomical site and extent, and size, shape and surface. Note the temperature and tenderness; raised temperature and positive tenderness will be found in strangulated hernia. The consistency is peculiar of the content; doughy in omentocele and elastic in enterocele. In suspected sports hernia, tenderness may be found on palpation over pubic symphysis and/or pubic tubercle and over superficial inguinal ring [7].

The test, "get above the lump", helps in differentiating a hernial swelling and a true scrotal swelling. The neck of the scrotum is hold on both sides, while feeling the structures in this area. If only the spermatic cords are felt and the swelling is below, it is true scrotal swelling. If the neck structures are thicker than the spermatic cord and the swelling is going up, it is either a hernia or congenital hydrocele. Gently pull the testis down, "traction test"; it may reveal encysted hydrocele of cord as it descends. Fluctuation and translucency tests will help in further defining the content of a scrotal hernial swelling and a true scrotal swelling like hematocele and hydrocele. The finger invagination test [5], consist of doctor invaginating his/her index finger into the canal through the root of scrotum and feeling the expansile impulse while the patient cough or do Valsalva maneuvers; however, I discourage performing this test as it is painful for the patients and doesn't add much to the diagnosis.

The final parts of palpation are done while the patient is lie down on the bed. The hernias with wide neck such as direct inguinal hernia or incisional hernia, usually reduces itself as the patient lie down. In long standing indirect inguinal hernia or paraumbilical, the patient usually knows how to reduce it. Ask them to reduce. If patient is unable to reduce, then ask to relax the abdominal muscles and hold the fundus of the sac, while applying constant gentle pressure, squeezing the contents towards the abdomen. The contents may reduce with gurgling (enterocele). Note the difficulty in reduction; in enterocele the first part is difficult to reduce but the last part goes in easily, while in omentocele first part reduces easily while the last part reduces with difficulty. However, in cases of complication like strangulation, a hernia can't be reduced. Never try to force reduction, as it may result in rupture of sac.

Ring occlusion test is a useful test to differentiate between a direct and an indirect inguinal hernia. The hernia must be reduced first. Begin by palpating the inguinal ligament and tracing it medially and laterally towards its bony attachments, pubic tubercle and anterior superior iliac spine, respectively. Locate the deep inguinal ring which lie 1.25 cm above the inguinal ligament midway between its two bony attachments. Occlude the deep inguinal ring with thumb and ask the patient to cough. If hernia comes out while the deep ring is occluded, it is direct inguinal hernia.

3-finger test is a similar test which helps in differentiating indirect inguinal, direct inguinal and femoral hernias. Here 3 rings are occluded simultaneously with 3 fingers; index finger on deep inguinal ring, middle finger on superficial inguinal ring (about 1.25 cm above the pubic tubercle) and ring finger over saphenous opening (about 4 cm below and lateral to pubic tubercle). The patient is asked to cough.

The expansile impulse at index finger indicates indirect inguinal hernia, middle finger indicates direct inguinal hernia and ring finger femoral hernia.

It is useful to examine the tone of abdominal muscles by asking to raise shoulders against resistance or lift both legs straight off the bed. This will also show a divarication of recti.

Finally, it is important to remember that local hernia examination must be supplemented by full abdominal and digital rectal examinations, as well as any other system if history is suggesting.

Author details

Muhammad Shamim
Department of Surgery, College of Medicine, Prince Sattam Bin Abdulaziz University, Saudi Arabia

*Address all correspondence to: surgeon.shamim@gmail.com

IntechOpen

References

[1] Light D, Chattopadhyay D, & Bawa S. Radiological and clinical examination in the diagnosis of Spigelian hernias. 2013; 98-100. https://doi.org/10.1308/003588 413X13511609957092

[2] Evers BM. Small bowel. In: Sabiston DC, Townsend CM, eds. Sabiston Textbook of Surgery: The Biological Basis of Modern Surgical Practice. 18th ed. Philadelphia, Pa.: Saunders/Elsevier; 2008:873-916.

[3] McIntosh A, Hutchinson A, Roberts A, Withers H. Evidence-based management of groin hernia in primary care—a systematic review. Fam Pract. 2000; 17(5):442-447.

[4] Kochupapy RT, Ranganathan G, Dias S, Shanahan D, & Hospital PP. Aetiology of femoral hernias revisited : bilateral femoral hernia in a young male (two cases). 2013; 14-16. https://doi.org/ 10.1308/003588413X13511609955733

[5] Leblanc KE, Leblanc LL, & Leblanc KA. Inguinal hernias: Diagnosis and management. American Family Physician. 2013

[6] Morelli V, Weaver V. Groin injuries and groin pain in athletes: part 1. Prim Care. 2005; 32(1):163-183.

[7] Brown A, Abrahams S, Remedios D, & Chadwick SJ. Clinical Intelligence Sports hernia : 2013 March; 235-237. https://doi.org/10.3399/bjgp13X664432

[8] van den Berg JC, de Valois JC, Go PM, Rosenbusch G. Detection of groin hernia with physical examination, ultrasound, and MRI compared with laparoscopic findings. Invest Radiol. 1999; 34(12):739-743.

Chapter 2

Minimally Invasive Surgery of the Groin: Inguinal Hernia Repair

César Felipe Ploneda-Valencia,

Carlos Alfredo Bautista-López,

Carlos Alberto Navarro-Montes

and Juan Carlos Verdugo-Tapia

Abstract

The minimally invasive surgical technique for inguinal hernia repair (eTEP and TAPP) are gaining acceptance among surgeons worldwide. With the superior benefits of the laparoendoscopic techniques (less postoperative pain, numbness, and chronic pain, fewer complications, and faster return to normal activities), the protocolization and standardization of these approaches are essential to improve patient outcomes and reduce costs. Improved laparoscopic skills, well-selected patients, simulator training, and anatomy knowledge of the groin are the cornerstone for these approaches. We recommend starting the learning curve with the TAPP procedure, because it is easier to get familiarized with the anatomical landmarks of the pelvis and groin.

Keywords: inguinal hernia, TAPP, TEP, E-TEP, minimally

1. Introduction

When dealing with groin hernia, we believe that surgeons must be familiarized with an open technique (Lichtenstein), a posterior open technique (e.g., Rives-Stoppa), a non-mesh technique (Shouldice or McVay), and a laparoendoscopic technique (TAPP or eTEP). The former is because the groin hernia has a lifetime occurrence of 27–43% in men and 3–6% in women [1]. Therefore, inguinal hernia repair (IHR) is one of the most common surgeries performed worldwide, doing approximately 20 million each year [2].

It is now well recognized that laparoendoscopic techniques are superior to open approaches concerning less postoperative pain, numbness [3], chronic pain, fewer complications, and faster return to normal activities [2–4]. Nevertheless, longer operative time, increased costs, and major complications such as great vessels and intestinal injuries are attributable to the laparoendoscopic approach [2–4]. Even though laparoendoscopic surgery is more expensive than open procedures [2], improved surgical skills, experienced surgeons, high-volume centers, and some patient characteristics (e.g., Bilateral inguinal hernia) enhance this approach [2, 4–6].

The minimally invasive surgical techniques for inguinal hernia repair (MISr): extended-view totally extraperitoneal approach (eTEP) and transabdominal preperitoneal approach (TAPP); are gaining ground in the surgeons' armamentarium.

Improved laparoscopic skills, well-selected patients, simulator training, and anatomy knowledge of the groin are the cornerstone for these approaches.

2. Anatomical considerations

The myopectineal orifice (MPO) is an inherently weak area of the abdominal wall where the direct, indirect, femoral, and oblique hernias occur [7], being delimited medially by rectus abdominis muscle, inferiorly by pectineus ligament, laterally by psoas muscle, and superiorly by the transverse arch (transversus abdominis and internal oblique muscle) [8]. The anatomical landmarks are described in **Figure 1**.

Two classic triangles have been described in the laparoscopic inguinal view: The triangle of doom (**Figure 2**) where the external iliac artery and vein are, and the triangle of pain (**Figure 2**), within this triangle, are from lateral to medial: the lateral femoral cutaneous nerve, the femoral branch of the genitofemoral nerve and the femoral nerve.

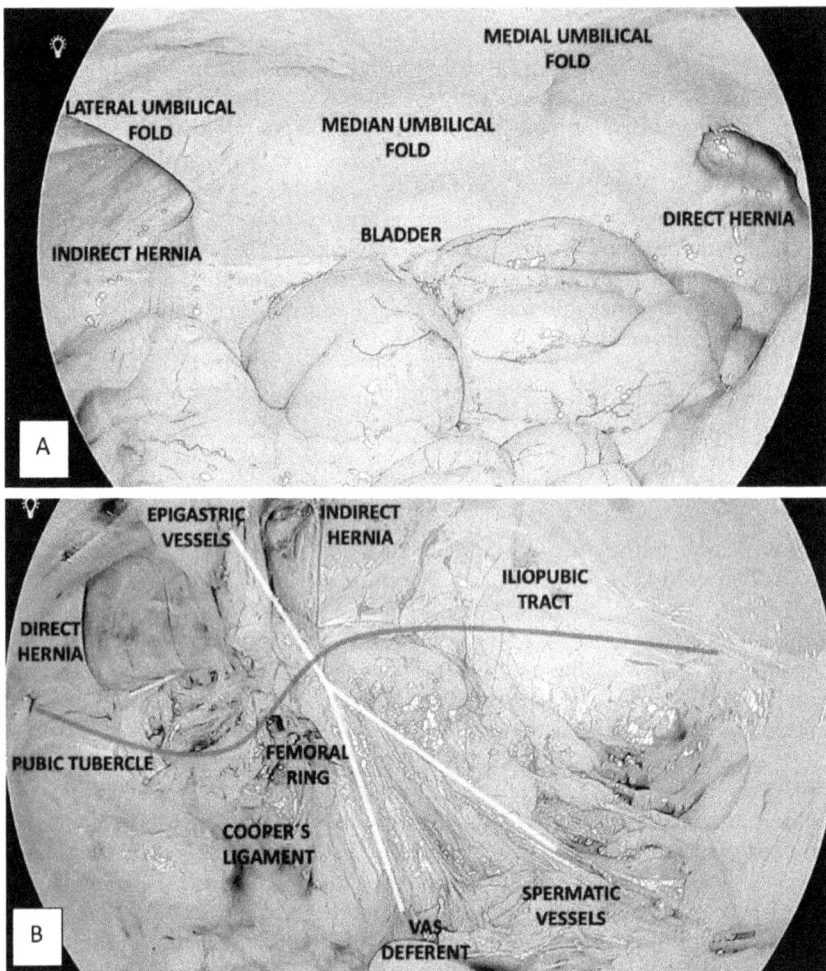

Figure 1.
Anatomical landmark of laparoscopic pelvic view (A) and inguinal laparoscopic view (B). Own by the author.

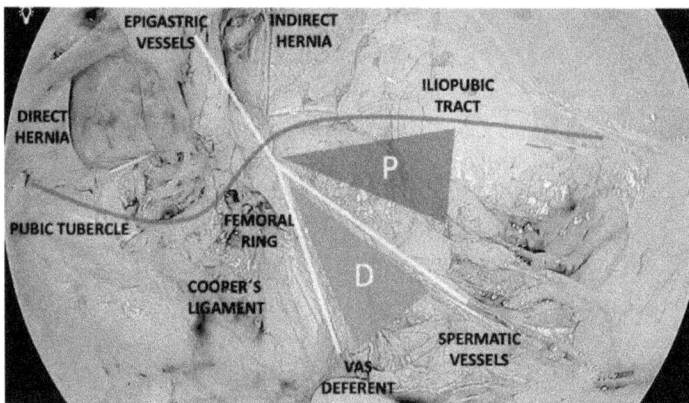

Figure 2.
Triangle of pain (P) and triangle of doom (D). Own by the author.

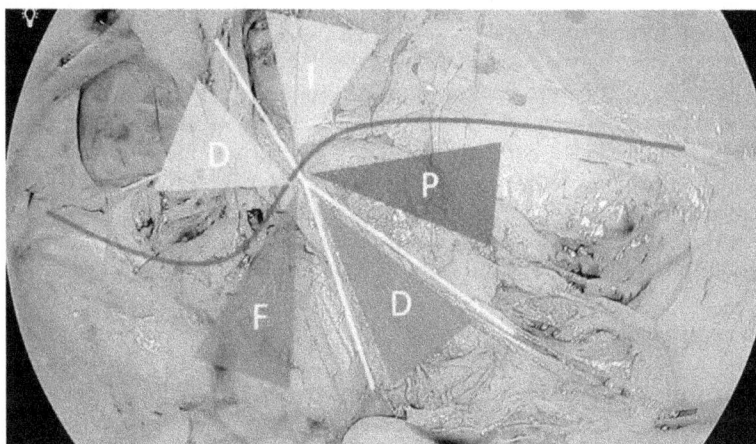

Figure 3.
Inverted "Y" and five triangles of the inguinal region. Femoral hernia (F), direct hernia (D), indirect hernia (I), doom (D) and pain (D) triangles. Own by the author.

A more didactic description of the MPO's posterior visualization dividing this region into three zones and five triangles was described to facilitate the comprehension and recognition of anatomical structures during MISr [8] (see **Figures 3** and **4**).

3. Surgical aspects

Even though the eTEP and the TAPP require a different initial approach, both techniques need to accomplish the MPO's critical view to assurance a correct mesh placement after the creation of the peritoneal pocket.

3.1 Indications and contraindications

The indications to perform a MISr of inguinal hernia are the same as those for an open approach. The more important indications to do MISr are: knowledge of the

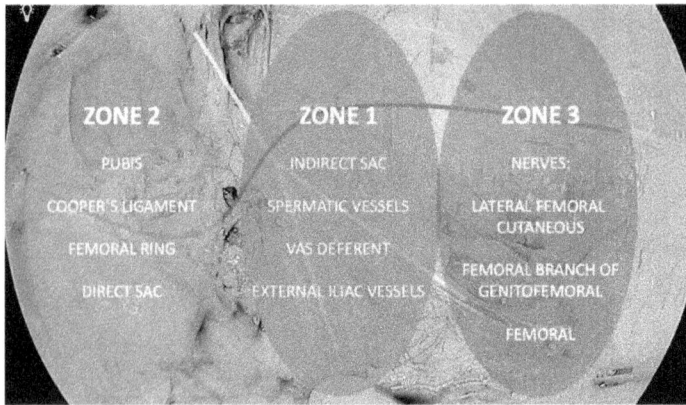

Figure 4.
Zones of the inguinal region. Own by the author.

technique with a clear laparoscopic anatomy concept, having laparoscopic skills for intracorporeal suture, and bimanual dissection capacity. In the case of an incarcerated or strangulated hernia, we recommend the TAPP approach to inspect the bowel; if small bowel resection must be done, intracorporeal stapler use or exteriorization of the bowel through the umbilical port (minilaparotomy of 5 cm) can be used.

The contraindications are the patient's intolerance to pneumoperitoneum, childhood, and pregnancy after the second trimester. Relative contraindications are severe ascites, strangulated hernia, recurrence inguinal hernia after a posterior approach.

As for the initial cases, we recommend starting with small, unilateral hernias and progressively, increase the difficulty of the cases.

3.2 Preoperative planning

Patient: patient's position on the operating table is supine with both arms secured at their respective side. Bladder drainage with a Foley catheter is unnecessary if the patient urinates immediately before entering the operating room; We suggest draining the bladder with a Foley catheter during the initial cases.

Instrument: laparoscopic tower, a 30 degrees 10 mm angular scope, two grasper or Croce-Olmi forceps, one Maryland dissector, one Metzenbaum scissors, one laparoscopic needle driver, monopolar energy.

The surgeon's position is on the hernia's contralateral side (Dr. Ploneda-Valencia usually operates at the patient's head). The camera's operator is on the hernia's side (or at the opposite of the hernia if the surgeon is at the patient's head). The operating table is kept in the Trendelenburg position with a contralateral rotation of the hernia. The monitor is placed at the patient's feet.

Comment: Our anesthetist usually applies a TAP block guided with ultrasound.

3.2.1 Standardize technique: critical view of the myopectineal orifice

The following are the steps to gain the critical view of the MPO, which are necessary to increase surgical success [9]:

1. Create a large peritoneal flap. Dissect across the midline and identify the pubic tubercle and Cooper's ligament (CL). For large, direct hernias, extend the dissection to the contralateral CL.

2. Rule out a direct hernia by visualizing the anatomy. Remove unusual fat in the Hesselbach's triangle.

3. Dissect the space of Retzius at least 2 cm between the CL and bladder to facilitate flat placement of the mesh.

4. Rule out a femoral hernia by dissecting between the CL and iliac vein.

5. Parietalize the cord's elements. To ensure compliance with this requirement, the dissection must continue until the cord's elements lie flat. Pull the sac and peritoneum upward; this maneuver will not trigger any movement of the cord's elements if this step is achieved.

6. Identify and reduce cord lipomas.

7. Dissect the peritoneum lateral to the cord's elements beyond the anterior superior iliac spine.

8. Perform the dissection and ensure that mesh provides adequate coverage of all defects. Mechanical fixation must be placed above an imaginary inter-anterior superior iliac spine line and any defects to avoid recurrence and nerve injury.

9. Place the mesh only when items 1 to 8 are completed, and hemostasis has been verified. The mesh size should be at least 15–10 cm and be placed without creases or folds. Ensure that its lateral-inferior corner lies deep against the wall and does not roll up during space deflation.

3.2.2 eTEP technical features

The initial incision is made on the flank 3 cm above and 5 cm lateral to the umbilicus line [6, 10, 11]. See **Figure 5** for unilateral hernia and **Figure 6** for bilateral hernia trocar setup. At the selected location, a 12 mm incision is made, and the anterior fascia is exposed with the use of "S" retractors, the anterior fascia is incised with a no. 11 blade, the fibers of the rectal abdominis muscle are separate, and the posterior sheath is exposed. Blunt dissection with the finger is done, and the space created is lifted with the help of the "S" retractor to allow the introduction of the balloon dissector (**Figure 7**). Once the balloon dissector (Spacemaker™ Plus Dissector System) is inserted, the camera is introduced, and the balloon is inflated with the hand pump with 25–30 hand pumps of air under direct vision. The next step should follow the critical view of the myopectineal orifice [9].

3.2.3 TAPP technical features

The trocar setup we recommend is demonstrated in **Figure 8**; the initial incision is transumbilical [12, 13], either Veress or Hasson technique can be done as the surgeons' preference, and a 12 mm trocar is introduced. After laparoscopy is done, two 5 mm trocar to the right and left of the umbilicus are introduced. Our recommendation for the peritoneal flap creation is to initiate the lateral side 2 cm upper and 2 cm medial to the anterior superior iliac spine. In a horizontal direction, it incises the peritoneum to the medial umbilical ligament (See **Figure 1**). The following dissection should be in a bloodless space, which could be done either in Zone 1 or in Zone 2 (See **Figure 4**). We recommend doing first the Zone 2 dissection because it

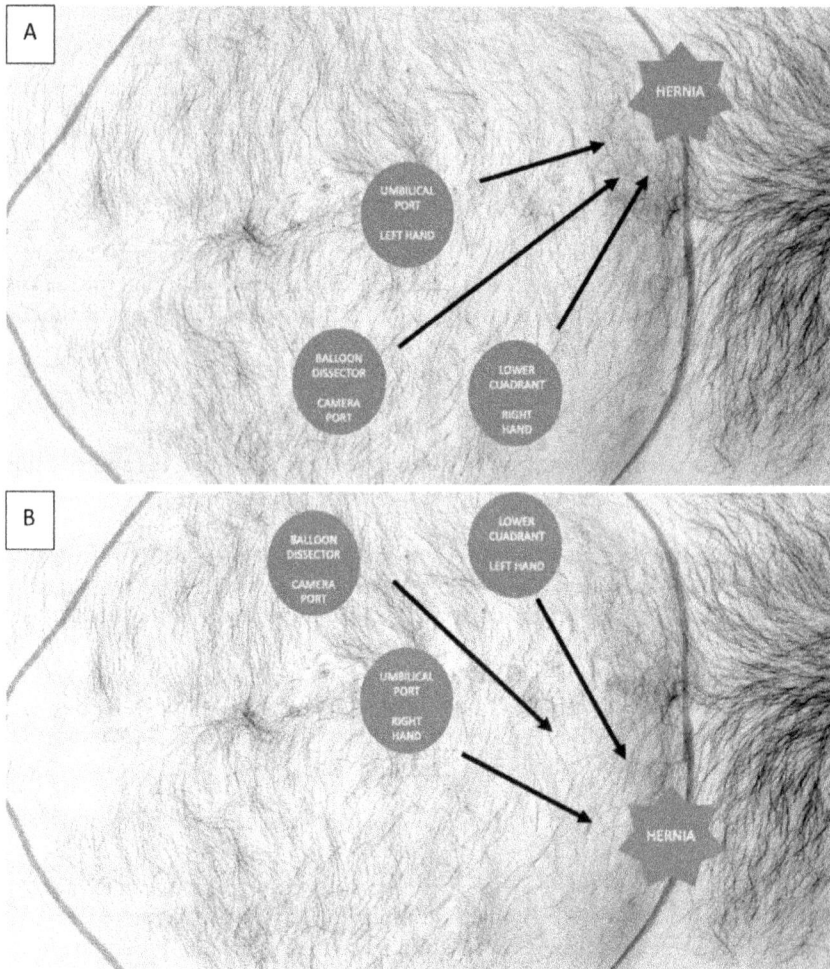

Figure 5.
eTEP for unilateral inguinal hernia trocar setup. "A" left hernia and "B" right hernia. Own by the author.

is easier to identify the CL and the pubic tubercle (**Figure 9**). The next step should follow the critical view of the myopectineal orifice [9].

3.2.4 Pitfalls and pearls

- The TAPP technique is easier to learn and has a more "friendly" view of the anatomical landmarks than eTEP.

- The dissection of Zone 2 is easier to do and has a more consistent anatomy.

- The medial defect should be close if it is larger than 2 cm. We recommend the use of the European Hernia Classification to describe the hernias [14].

- The lateral hernia sac should be traction medially. Remember, "traction" and "counteraction" are the key steps to dissect the sac.

- "Twist" medially the sac to improve the traction.

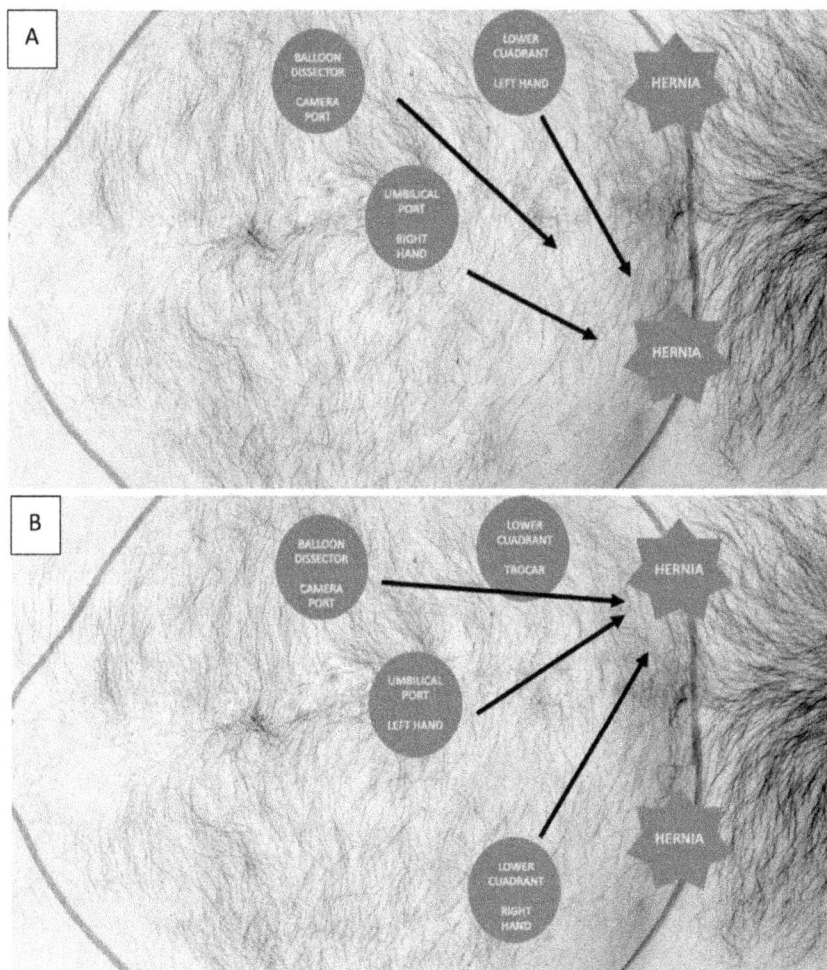

Figure 6.
eTEP bilateral inguinal hernia trocar setup. "A" start with the right hernia; "B" insert a fourth trocar in the rigth lower cuadrant to do the left hernia.

- The dissection of the cord's elements is achieved when we tract the peritoneal flap, and the movement is not transmitted to the cord's elements; the sac must reach the peritoneal flap.

- In larger sacs, the "ligation and section" approach is a valid option

- If bleeding from the "Corona Mortis" occurs, simple compression with two or three gauzes is usually enough for 5 to 10 minutes. We do not recommend using electrocautery as it may tear the vessel or increase the zone of bleeding.

- The mesh should be at least 12 cm transversely and 11 cm vertically. We usually use a 14×14 cm mesh.

- We do not recommend using a pre-shaped mesh because it only increases the cost of the procedure. We use a polypropylene mesh of 15×15 cm (Ultrapro™ or Prolene™) and cut it to fix. We only cut the border of the mesh. See **Figure 10**

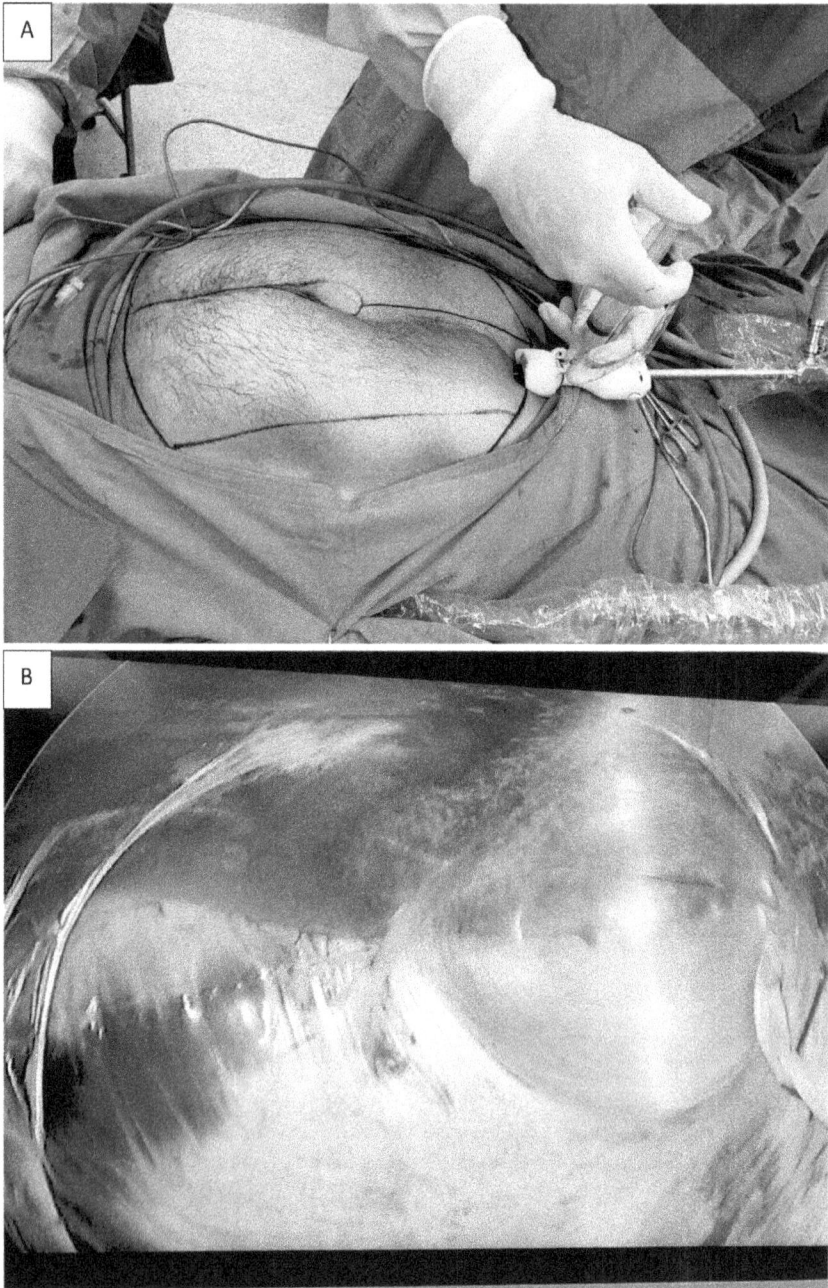

Figure 7.
Balloon dissector outside (A) and inside (B) view of the abdomen. Own by the author.

- We recommend rolling up the mesh to introduce the mesh and place an external stitch to maintain the position. Once inside, cut the stitch and unroll it, pulling the mesh's inferior medial aspect downward and unrolling upward. See **Figure 11**

- To fix the mesh, either use 1–2 Tackers in CL, 1 Tacker medial, and 1 Tacker lateral and in the most upper part of the mesh to avoid the triangle of pain or use

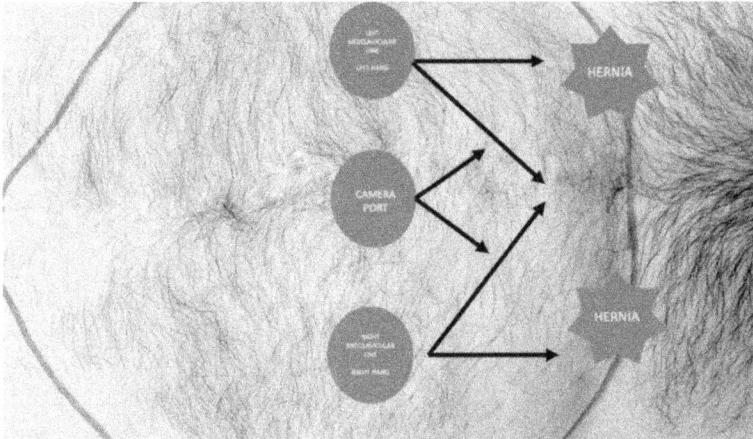

Figure 8.
TAPP trocar setup. Own by the author.

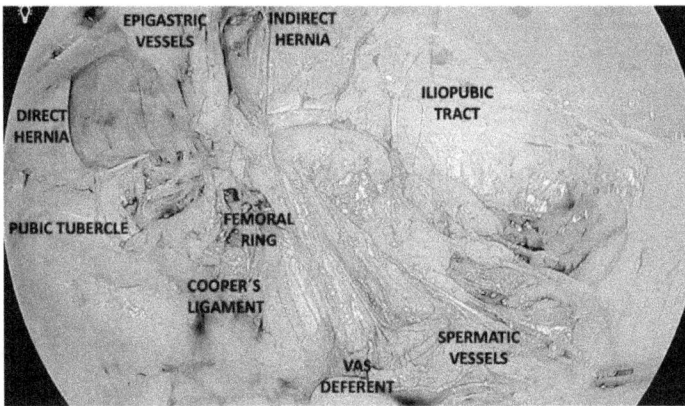

Figure 9.
Complete inguinal dissection. Own by the author.

absorbable stitches instead. Always remember not to apply it over the inferior epigastric vessels or beneath an imaginary line that runs transversely from the iliopubic tract to the pubic tubercle (See **Figure 3**). See **Figure 12**.

- Even though experts do not fix the mesh [15], we strongly recommend fixing it to diminish migration risk. On the other hand, the mesh's excessive fixation won't prevent a recurrence if the surgical technique isn't performed correctly and will increase the risk of postoperative pain and chronic pain [16].

- Tears can appear during the creation of the peritoneal flap, making it complicated to cover the mesh. Using the redundant peritoneal sac to cover the mesh with peritoneum is a feasible option.

3.2.5 Postoperative care

In the small or medium-sized hernias (L/M < 3), we managed the patient as an outpatient; during the learning curve, a 12–24 hours observation may be advisable.

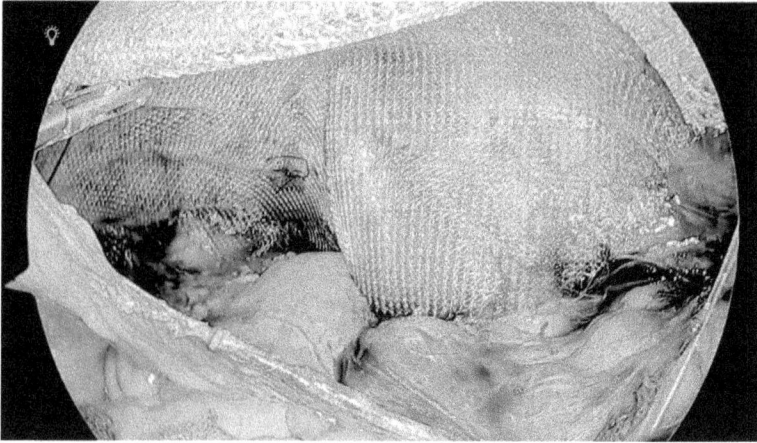

Figure 10.
Mesh configuration. Own by the author.

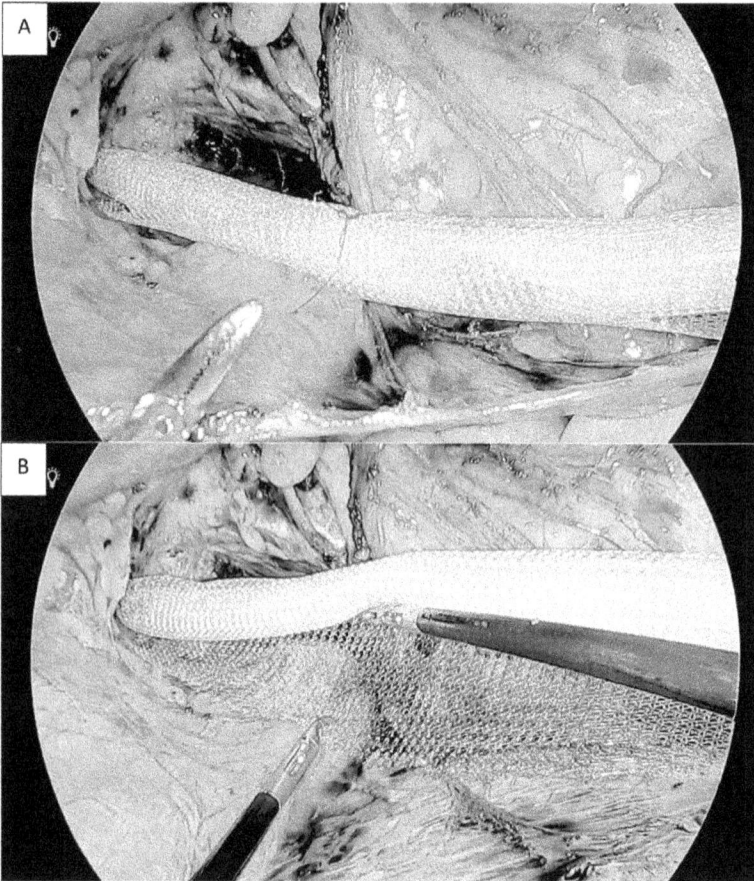

Figure 11.
Roll up mesh (A) and unroll the mesh from downward to upward (B). Own by the author.

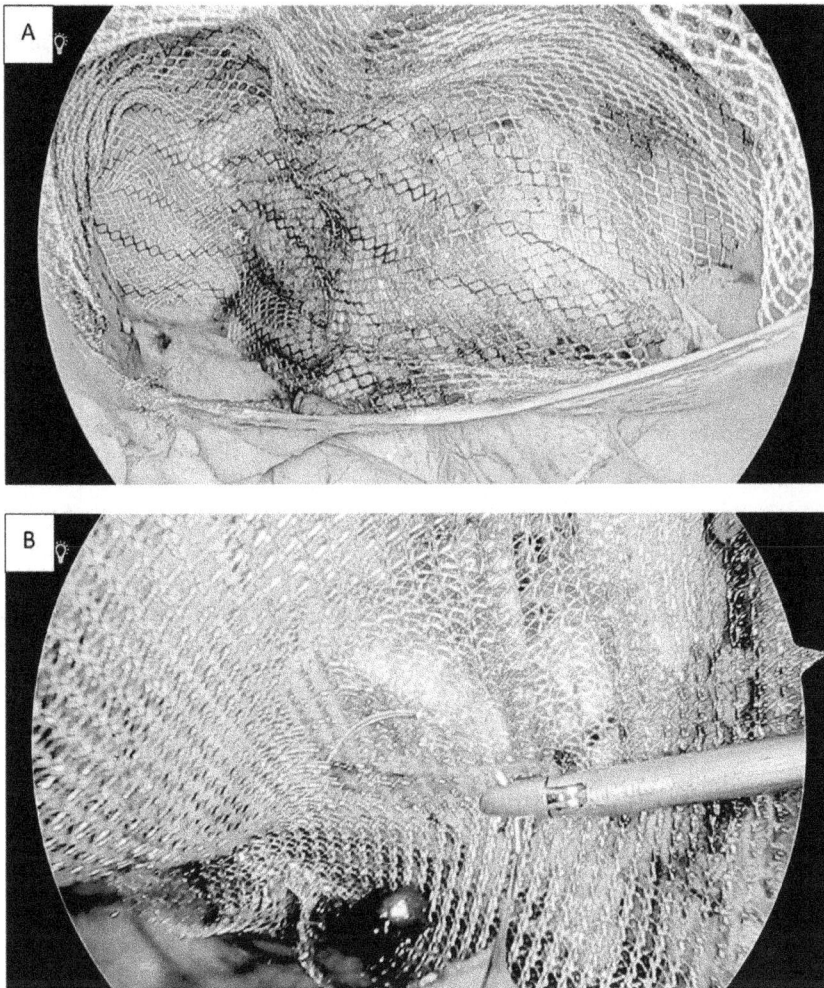

Figure 12.
Fix mesh either with tackers (A) or stitches (B). Own by the author.

The use of tight boxers and an icepack application in the groin region reduces postoperative pain and the inflammatory response. We recommend using the icepack for 30 minutes four times a day during the first seven days. Physical activity, mild activities (such as driving or going to work) are recommended after the 7th postoperative day; lifting over 10 kg or doing exercise is recommended after the 4th postoperative week.

3.3 Complications

Transoperative complications: the most common complication is peritoneal flap tear, which can be closed with the remanent sac or by diminishing the insufflator's pressure to do a primary closure. Bleeding of large vessels is a life-threatening complication. The more frequent injured vessels are the inferior epigastric vessels or the obturator vessels. If bleeding occurs, compression with gauze for

10 minutes is usually enough; using titanium clips or an advanced hemostatic device (LigasureTM or HarmonicTM) may resolve the problem. The surgeon must be ready to convert the surgery if the bleeding is abundant. As for the intestinal lesion, the surgeon's ability to do a primary closure with intracorporeal suture will decide the course of action. If the surgical field is contaminated, an open non-mesh technique should be done.

Postoperative complications include pain, seroma, hematoma, hydrocele, surgical site infection, chronic pain, mesh rejection, mesh infection, recurrence, testicular atrophy, among other less common complications (e.g., mesh penetration of the bladder). Seroma is the most frequent complication, usually appears in a large hernia, secondary either to death-space or to an exhaustive dissection of a large sac. Hematoma is another frequent complication which diminishes its appearance if tight boxers and icepack on the groin are used. Generally, watchful waiting is enough to manage either seroma or hematoma, but surgical drainage may be needed if large and painful.

4. Conclusions

MISr is safe and feasible if the surgeon is familiarized with the anatomical landmarks and the technique. Surgical skills and experience are essential to improve patient outcomes. Reviewing the surgery video, especially during the learning curve or in complicated cases, and comparing it with the expert's videos, enhances the surgeon's growth and diminishes the learning curve.

Conflict of interest

The authors declare no conflict of interest.

Author details

César Felipe Ploneda-Valencia[1*], Carlos Alfredo Bautista-López[2], Carlos Alberto Navarro-Montes[1] and Juan Carlos Verdugo-Tapia[1]

1 CEMIJAL (Cirugía Endoscópica y de Mínima Invasión Jalisco), CHG Hospital, Guadalajara, Jalisco, México

2 Hospital Civil de Guadalajara "Dr. Juan I. Menchaca", Guadalajara, Jalisco, México

*Address all correspondence to: dr.ploneda.cirugia@gmail.com

IntechOpen

References

[1] The HerniaSurge Group. International guidelines for groin hernia management. Hernia. febrero de 2018;22(1):1-165.

[2] Tadaki C, Lomelin D, Simorov A, Jones R, Humphreys M, daSilva M, et al. Perioperative outcomes and costs of laparoscopic versus open inguinal hernia repair. Hernia. junio de 2016;20(3):399-404.

[3] Cavazzola LT, Rosen MJ. Laparoscopic Versus Open Inguinal Hernia Repair. Surg Clin North Am. octubre de 2013;93(5):1269-1279.

[4] Pisanu A, Podda M, Saba A, Porceddu G, Uccheddu A. Meta-analysis and review of prospective randomized trials comparing laparoscopic and Lichtenstein techniques in recurrent inguinal hernia repair. Hernia. junio de 2015;19(3):355-366.

[5] Ielpo B, Nuñez-Alfonsel J, Duran H, Diaz E, Fabra I, Caruso R, et al. Cost-effectiveness of Randomized Study of Laparoscopic Versus Open Bilateral Inguinal Hernia Repair: Ann Surg. noviembre de 2018;268(5):725-730.

[6] Daes J. Minimally Invasive Surgical Techniques for Inguinal Hernia Repair: The Extended-View Totally Extraperitoneal Approach (eTEP). En: Davis, SS, Dakin G, Bates A, editores. The SAGES Manual of Hernia Surgery [Internet]. Cham: Springer International Publishing; 2019 [citado 22 de noviembre de 2020]. p. 449-60. Disponible en: http://link.springer.com/10.1007/978-3-319-78411-3_33

[7] Yang X-F, Liu J-L. Anatomy essentials for laparoscopic inguinal hernia repair. Ann Transl Med. octubre de 2016;4(19):372-372.

[8] Furtado M, Claus CMP, Cavazzola LT, Malcher F, Bakonyi-Neto A, Saad-Hossne R. Systemization of laparoscopic inguinal hernia repair (tapp) based on a new anatomical concept: inverted y and five triangles. ABCD Arq Bras Cir Dig São Paulo. 2019;32(1):e1426.

[9] Daes J, Felix E. Critical View of the Myopectineal Orifice: Ann Surg. julio de 2017;266(1):e1-e2.

[10] Claus C, Furtado M, Malcher F, Cavazzola LT, Felix E. Ten golden rules for a safe MIS inguinal hernia repair using a new anatomical concept as a guide. Surg Endosc. abril de 2020;34(4):1458-1464.

[11] Daes J. The enhanced view–totally extraperitoneal technique for repair of inguinal hernia. Surg Endosc. abril de 2012;26(4):1187-1189.

[12] Inga-Zapata E, García F. MIS Techniques: Lap TAPP and rTAPP. En: Davis, SS, Dakin G, Bates A, editores. The SAGES Manual of Hernia Surgery [Internet]. Cham: Springer International Publishing; 2019 [citado 22 de noviembre de 2020]. p. 415-27. Disponible en: http://link.springer.com/10.1007/978-3-319-78411-3_30

[13] Garcia-Ruiz A, Weber-Sanchez A. Laparoscopic Transabdominal Preperitoneal Inguinal Hernia Repair. En: Fischer JE, Jones DB, editores. Master Techniques in Surgery Hernia. Philadelphia PA: Lippincott Williams & Williams, Wolter Kluwer; 2013. p. 161-72.

[14] Miserez M, Alexandre JH, Campanelli G, Corcione F, Cuccurullo D, Pascual MH, et al. The European hernia society groin hernia classication: simple and easy to remember. Hernia. 22 de marzo de 2007;11(2):113-6.

[15] Palmisano EM, Aguilar Ruiz MJ. Transabdominal pre-peritoneal inguinal

hernioplasty (TAPP) without mesh fixation. Initial experience in the short term. Rev Hispanoam Hernia [Internet]. 2019 [citado 23 de noviembre de 2020]; Disponible en: https://hernia.grupoaran. com/articles/00234/show

[16] Yheulon C, Davis SS. Fixation vs. No Fixation in MIS Inguinal Hernia Repair. En: Davis, SS, Dakin G, Bates A, editores. The SAGES Manual of Hernia Surgery [Internet]. Cham: Springer International Publishing; 2019 [citado 23 de noviembre de 2020]. p. 391-5. Disponible en: http://link.springer. com/10.1007/978-3-319-78411-3_28

Chapter 3

Femoral Hernia: Open and Laparoscopic Surgery Approaches

Muhammad Shamim

Abstract

Femoral hernia comes out of abdominal cavity through the femoral canal and descends vertically to saphenous opening, and once escapes this opening it expands considerably, sometimes rising above the inguinal ligament. Due to its tortuous course, the hernia is usually irreducible and liable to strangulate. There are different open surgery choices. In low (Lockwood) operation, the sac is dissected out below the inguinal ligament via a groin-crease incision. In high (McEvedy) operation, the hernia is accessed via a horizontal (or vertical) incision made in lower abdomen at the lateral edge of rectus muscle. In Lotheissen's operation, the hernia is approached through the inguinal canal. The last one is my preferred approach, as it also helps in dealing if the contents are strangulated. The laparoscopic approaches include both transabdominal preperitoneal repair (TAPP) and total extraperitoneal repair (TEP). This chapter will give an account of the advantages and disadvantages of these different surgical techniques.

Keywords: Hernia, femoral, surgery approaches, surgical techniques

1. Introduction

Femoral hernia is protrusion of a part of abdominal viscus or preperitoneal fat through the femoral ring and canal. The canal forms the most medial compartment of femoral sheath, and extends from femoral ring above to saphenous opening below. The boundaries of femoral ring and canal consists of inguinal ligament (anteriorly), lacunar ligament (medially), thin septum (laterally), and iliopectineal ligament, pubic bone and pectineal fascia (posteriorly). Usually, the canal contains some fat, few lymphatics and lymph node of Cloquet.

The hernia first descends vertically down to saphenous opening, and once out of the opening, it expands considerably, sometimes rising above the inguinal ligament, assuming a retort-like shape. Because of its narrow course in the femoral canal and tortuous course after escaping saphenous opening, it is liable to become irreducible and strangulate. Sometimes, the neck of the sac become plugged with omentum or adhesions, and the empty sac filled with fluid resulting in hydrocele. Sometimes, instead of coming via femoral ring, it comes through a gap in lacunar ligament, and nearly always strangulate.

2. Clinical presentation

Femoral hernia accounts for less than 5% of all abdominal wall hernias and is more common in females than males (4:1) [1–3]. It usually develop after puberty, with increased incidence between 20 and 40 years. The patients usually present with a groin lump with some pain and discomfort (due to narrow and tortuous course). Incarceration is more common in femoral hernia due to narrow neck of femoral canal, and omental/bowel strangulation is associated with higher morbidity and mortality [3–5]. Patients with obstruction/strangulation of small bowel usually presents with colicky abdominal pain, distension, vomiting and constipation. On examination, the hernia is found below and lateral to pubic tubercle but once it escapes from saphenous opening it can spread in any direction and may be found above the inguinal ligament. The cough impulse is usually absent, even in uncomplicated cases, due to narrow neck and adhesions. The sac is usually occupied by omentum (dull note and firm consistency), or it remains empty being surrounded by extra-peritoneal fat [4]. However, it may contain bowel as well (resonant note and soft consistency). The rare reported contents include appendix (De Garengeot's hernia), bladder, Meckle's diverticulum, ectopic testis, stomach and fallopian tube [6–8].

3. Diagnostic imaging

Clinical diagnosis requires a high index of suspicion but it usually remain inconclusive. The ultrasonography, computed tomography and magnetic resonance imaging help in identifying doubtful cases [6, 9]. It can help in preoperative diagnosis of complications like the presence of appendicitis within femoral hernial sac [2].

4. Treatment

Elective repair should be undertaken once the diagnosis is made because of the risk of strangulation (due to narrow neck, tortuous course and adhesions). The reported obstruction/strangulation rate in literature is 30–86%, with mortality rates of 10–14% [10–12]. Emergency surgery with intestinal resections may be required in 9.3–33.7%, with a high mortality rate of 4.9% [4, 13, 14]. The hernia repair can be done by different open or laparoscopic approaches, with some advantages and disadvantages of each method. The choice is also affected by surgeon's preference, patient condition and elective/emergency condition.

5. Open surgical repair

5.1 Femoral (low, Lockwood's) approach

This is a simple and quick approach [1, 15] to deal with a small uncomplicated femoral hernia, and can be performed under local anesthesia. A transverse groin-crease incision is made below the inguinal ligament to dealt with the sac and its coverings. The content, usually omentum, is freed of adhesions and assessed for viability and either return back or excised. If necessary, a small incision can be made in lacunar ligament medially to ease reduction; however, abnormal branch of obturator artery can be injured. The neck is pulled down and ligated as high as possible. Finally, the canal is closed by suturing inguinal ligament to iliopectineal line using prolene 0 or 2/0 sutures; a mesh plug can also be used to close the defect.

5.2 Inguinal (Lotheissen's) approach

This is an easy approach as [1, 15] most of the steps are similar to that of open inguinal hernia repair. This should be the preferred approach in cases of complicated femoral hernia as it provides good exposure of femoral ring and facilitates in dealing with non-viable contents that necessitates resection. This approach also allows easy control of injured abnormal obturator artery. Inguinal canal is opened by giving an incision about 1.25 cm above the medial two-thirds of inguinal ligament, and incising external oblique aponeurosis in line of its fibers. The cord is mobilized and retracted upward, and blunt dissections are made to reach the transversalis fascia, which is opened medial to epigastric vessels from deep inguinal ring to pubic tubercle. The femoral hernia lies below this incision, which is reduced by both pulling from above and pushing from below. The peritoneum can be opened to help in reduction. The content is assessed for viability and dealt accordingly. In cases of obstruction at the narrow neck of the sac, the neck can be gently stretched with a hemostat. The neck is then closed with sutures or mesh plug. The defect is closed by suturing the conjoint tendon to ilio-pectineal line, so as to form a shutter. The layers of inguinal canal are then closed. The classical McVay repair (suturing conjoint tendon to Cooper's ligament) is strong but with high tension which eventually break resulting in recurrence [9].

5.3 Preperitoneal (high, McEvedy's) approach

This is the best approach [1, 15] in emergency setting to deal with bowel strangulation as it allows generous incision in peritoneum to give proper exposure for bowel resection [15]. A horizontal (or vertical) incision is made in lower abdomen at the lateral edge of rectus muscle. Anterior rectus sheath is incised and rectus muscle retracted medially. Dissection is carried out deep to this muscle in the preperitoneal space. The femoral hernia is delivered and its sac opened to assess the viability of contents, which is then dealt accordingly. The sac is first closed and the defect is then closed with sutures, mesh or plug. Placement of mesh in preperitoneal space is advantageous, as it avoids reoperating through scar tissue in cases of recurrence [16]. The mesh-plug repair offers tension free easy repairs, with low recurrence rate and less postoperative pain [3, 5].

6. Laparoscopic surgery

The laparoscopic surgery offers the advantages of minimal access surgery including excellent exposure, identification of occult hernia, reduce postoperative pain and faster recuperation [6]. The TEP laparoscopic approach is suitable for uncomplicated femoral hernia, while for incarcerated or strangulated hernia TAPP approach can be used.

6.1 Transabdominal preperitoneal (TAPP) approach

The theater setup, patient position and port placements are as described in chapter 3 (Laparoscopic inguinal hernia repair by Dr. Ploneda). The surgeon positions on the contralateral side. We usually create pneumoperitoneum using open first port technique. After insufflation, the patient is placed in Trendelenburg position to displace bowels up away from the dissection site. The key anatomical landmarks are identified (Figures 1–4, chapter 3) including femoral ring and deep inguinal ring, as well as medial umbilical ligament, inguinal ligament, bony landmarks (pubic tubercle and anterior superior iliac spine), vessels (epigastric, spermatic and iliac) and vas deferens. The opposite inguino-femoral areas are also visualized to identify any undiagnosed hernia.

The peritoneum is incised transversely above the deep inguinal ring extending from anterior superior iliac spine to medial umbilical ligament. The lower peritoneal flap is dissected to expose the hernial defects, inguinal ligament and Cooper's ligament. The hernial sac is identified and dissected carefully, avoiding injury to inferior epigastric vessels, iliac vessels and cord. If present, inguinal hernia is dealt at the same time. The peritoneal incision can be extended circumferentially to incise the neck of the sac leaving the distal sac in place (of a large hernial sac). A small hernial sac is left intact and pulled into the peritoneal cavity.

A large mesh (12 x 15 cm) is placed covering the entire inguino-femoral hernial orifices, and fixed either with staples or sutures to the pubic tubercle, medial end of Cooper's ligament and rectus muscle. The peritoneum is then closed with sutures or staples. The port sites are then closed.

6.2 Total extra-peritoneal (TEP) approach

The inguino-femoral hernia orifices are approached by creating extraperitoneal space by CO_2, so as to decrease the morbidity associated with peritoneal approach. This gives wide access to both inguino-femoral regions at the same time; however, the approach is not suitable if patient have had some previous surgery in this area. A small (1–2 cm) incision is made just below the umbilicus and blunt dissection is carried out to rectus sheath, which is then incised longitudinally to expose peritoneum or posterior rectus sheath. Care is taken not to open the peritoneum. A working space is created with dissecting balloon. The hernial sac is identified which is dealt, followed by repair of the defect (as described for TAPP).

7. Postoperative complications

In addition to the general complications of surgery, anesthesia and pneumoperitoneum, the specific procedure related complication can happen. The complication rate of over 50% have been reported in patients with intestinal resection [17]. These include dissection or stapling injury to iliofemoral vessels, epigastric vessels, spermatic vessels, vas, lateral femoral cutaneous nerve and femoral nerve. Other complications include wound seroma or hematoma, inguino-scrotal edema, hematoma or emphysema, bladder injury and bowel adhesion to mesh [9, 18]. Most of these complications are avoided by gentle and careful dissection under vision. Femoral hernia repair is more liable for recurrence than inguinal hernia repair, and the recurrence is more with sutures repair than with the use of synthetic patch/ mesh [9, 19]. Neurovascular and visceral injuries were reported more common with non-mesh repairs, whereas wound infection was more common with mesh repair [9].

Author details

Muhammad Shamim
Department of Surgery, College of Medicine, Prince Sattam Bin Abdulaziz
University, Alkharj, Saudi Arabia

*Address all correspondence to: surgeon.shamim@gmail.com

IntechOpen

References

[1] Pillay Y. Laparoscopic repair of an incarcerated femoral hernia. Int J Surg Case Rep [Internet]. 2015; 17:85-8. Available from: doi:10.1016/j.ijscr.2015.10.031

[2] Papatheofani V, Estaller W, Hoffmann TF. Femoral hernia with vermiform appendix herniation: a case report and review of the literature. J Surg Case Reports. 2021;2021(3):1-2.

[3] Clyde DR, de Beaux A, Tulloh B, O'Neill JR. Minimising recurrence after primary femoral hernia repair; is mesh mandatory? Hernia [Internet]. 2020;24(1):137-42. Available from: doi:10.1007/s10029-019-02007-6

[4] Gonzalez-Urquijo M, Tellez-Giron VC, Martinez-Ledesma E, Rodarte-Shade M, Estrada-Cortinas OJ, Gil-Galindo G. Bowel obstruction as a serious complication of patients with femoral hernia. Surg Today [Internet]. 2021;51(5):738-44. Available from: doi:10.1007/s00595-020-02158-5

[5] Aksoy F. Open-tension free three-dimensional Cooper ligament repair for femoral hernia. Asian J Surg [Internet]. 2018;41(2):183-6. Available from: doi:10.1016/j.asjsur.2016.11.006

[6] Alkashty M, Dickinson B, Tebala GD. Coloproctology De Garengeot' s Hernia Treated With a Hybrid Approach: A Case Report. 2021;21-23.

[7] Alzaraa A. Unusual Contents of the Femoral Hernia. ISRN Obstet Gynecol. 2011; 2011:1-2.

[8] P. Marioni, "Metastatic carcinoma with small intestine in a femoral hernia," Canadian Medical Association Journal, vol. 82, pp. 1081-1082, 1960.

[9] Lockhart K, Dunn D, Teo S, Ng JY, Dhillon M, Teo E, et al. Mesh versus non-mesh for inguinal and femoral hernia repair. Cochrane Database Syst Rev. 2018;2018(9).

[10] Kulah B, Duzgun AP, Moran M, Kulacoglu IH, Ozmen MM, Coskun F: Emergency Hernia Repairs in Elderly Patients. Am J Surg 2001, 182(5): 455-459.

[11] Kingsnorth A, LeBlanc K. Hernias: inguinal and incisional hernias. Lancet. 2003;362:1561e1571.

[12] Waddington RT. Femoral hernia, a recent appraisal. Br J Surg. 1971;58: 920e922.

[13] Humes DJ, Radcliffe RS, Camm C et al (2013) Population-based study of presentation and adverse outcomes after femoral hernia surgery. Br J Surg 100:1827-1832. doi:10.1002/bjs.9336

[14] Derici H, Unalp HR, Bozdag AD et al (2007) Factors affecting morbidity and mortality in incarcerated abdominal wall hernias. Hernia 11:341-346. https ://doi.org/10.1007/s1002 9-007-0226-3

[15] Sorelli PG, El-Masry NS, Garrett W V. Open femoral hernia repair: One skin incision for all. World J Emerg Surg. 2009;4(1):3-5.

[16] Karatepe O, Acet E, Altiok M, Adas G, Cakir A, Karahan S. Preperitoneal repair (open posterior approach) for recurrent inguinal hernias previously treated with Lichtenstein tension-free hernioplasty. Hippokratia. 2010;14:119e121.

[17] Cakir M, Savas OA, Tuzun S, Tatar C. Preperitoneal Mesh Placement with Anterior Approach in Incarcerated Femoral Hernia (Our Experiences with 23 Cases). Haseki Tip Bülteni 2015;53:196-198.

[18] Jiang XM, Sun RX, Huang WH, Yu JP. Midline preperitoneal repair for incarcerated and strangulated femoral hernia. Hernia [Internet]. 2019;23(2): 323-8. Available from: doi:10.1007/s10029-018-1848-3

[19] Dahlstrand U, Wollert S, Nordin P, Sandblom G, Gunnarsson U. Emergency femoral hernia repair: a study based on a national register. Ann Surg 2009;249: 672-676.

Chapter 4

Umbilical Hernias in Adults: Epidemiology, Diagnosis and Treatment

*Ibrahima Konaté, Abdourahmane Ndong
and Jacques N. Tendeng*

Abstract

The literature on umbilical hernias in adults remains less extensive compared to other types of hernias. Adult umbilical hernias are frequently asymptomatic. The most frequent reasons for consultation are pain and esthetic discomfort. The diagnosis is most often evident on physical examination of the abdomen with tumefaction in the umbilicus. Despite the recent advances in terms of mesh varieties and minimally invasive surgery (laparoscopic and robotic surgery), there is still no real consensus on the optimal method for repair of umbilical hernia. Based on the patient characteristics and the context, "tailored and optimized surgery" should always be used to have the best results.

Keywords: umbilicus, hernia, adult, abdominal wall, surgery

1. Introduction

An umbilical hernia is defined as a midline hernia located at or near the umbilicus [1]. Umbilicus is a frequent site of hernia because it represents a natural weak spot of the abdominal wall, being the attachment site of the umbilical cord during the fetal period.

The literature on umbilical hernias in adults remains less extensive compared to other types of hernias. In fact, in adults, groin hernias are more frequent, since umbilical hernias are more studied in children.

The risk of strangulation is important, estimated at up to 17% in umbilical hernias, up to three times higher than in femoral hernia [2]. To avoid these complications, a surgical treatment is required. Despite the recent advances in terms of mesh varieties and minimally invasive surgery (laparoscopic and robotic surgery), there is still no consensus on the optimal method for repair of umbilical hernia.

2. Epidemiology

It is estimated that every year, 20 million abdominal wall hernias surgeries are performed worldwide [3]. Umbilical hernia is the second most frequent type of hernia and accounts for 6–14% of all abdominal wall hernias in adults, after inguinal hernias [1].

It is a very common condition in children, occurring in one of every six children [4]. It represents an important part in the practice of pediatric surgeons, especially in sub-Saharan Africa [5]. However, in adults, nearly 90% of umbilical hernias are acquired with no indication of hernia in childhood [6]. The risk factors are the same as for other abdominal wall hernias and are caused predominantly by intra-abdominal hyper pressure and/or parietal weakness. The repetitive action on the abdominal wall due to increased intraabdominal pressure favor microscopic tears of tissue. This will lead in time to hernia formation.

The risk factors are physical labor, obesity, ascites, constipation, pregnancies, excessive coughing, or dysuria. A female predominance is however noted with a sex ratio of 3:1 [7]. This is explained by the different distribution of risk factors according to sex. Indeed, obesity is more common in women and pregnancy is a factor noted exclusively in women. This female predominance is also due to the distension of the umbilicus associated with childbirth.

3. Diagnosis

3.1 Clinical presentation

Umbilical hernias occur more often above or below the umbilicus rather than directly through the umbilicus [8]. This is why, according to the classification of the European Hernia Society, hernias whose rings are located between 3 cm on either side of the umbilicus on the linea alba, are considered as umbilical hernias (**Figure 1**) [9].

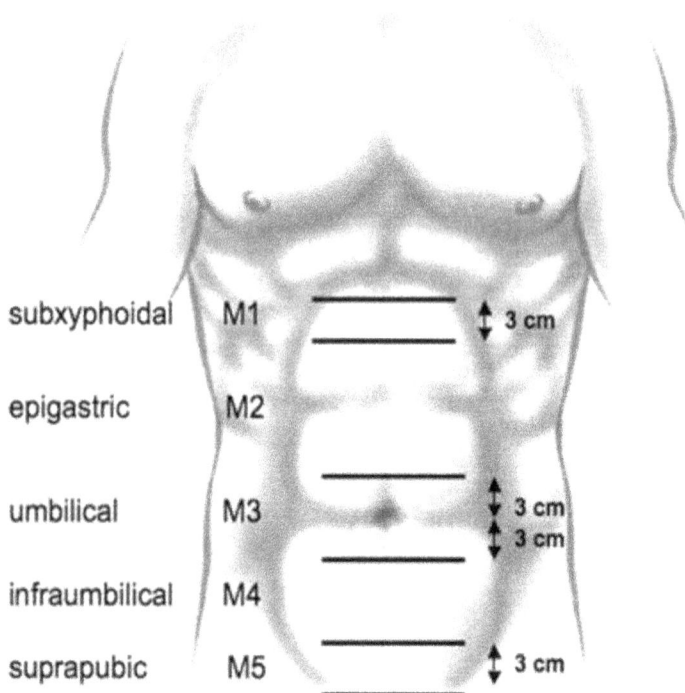

Figure 1.
Localization of umbilical hernias according to the classification of the European hernia society [9].

Adult umbilical hernias are frequently asymptomatic. The most frequent reasons for consultation are intermittent pain and esthetic discomfort when the size is important [2].

Palpation helps assess the size of the neck and the reducibility of the hernia. When there is a complication, the abdominal pain is constant. The main complication is strangulation (occurrence of ischemia due to a compromised blood supply). In most cases, patients with a strangulated hernia have previously experienced incarceration seizures with spontaneous reduction.

On physical examination, palpation reveals an irreducible and painful umbilical swelling. **Figure 2** shows a strangulated umbilical hernia with irreducible swelling. When the small intestines are in the hernia sac, signs of intestinal obstruction appear (vomiting, lack of gas or stool).

Another complication that can occur is loss of domain. It represents a chronic large irreducible hernia reducing the volume of the abdominal cavity and creating a "second abdomen" [10].

The diagnosis of umbilical hernia is most often evident on physical examination of the abdomen with tumefaction in the umbilicus.

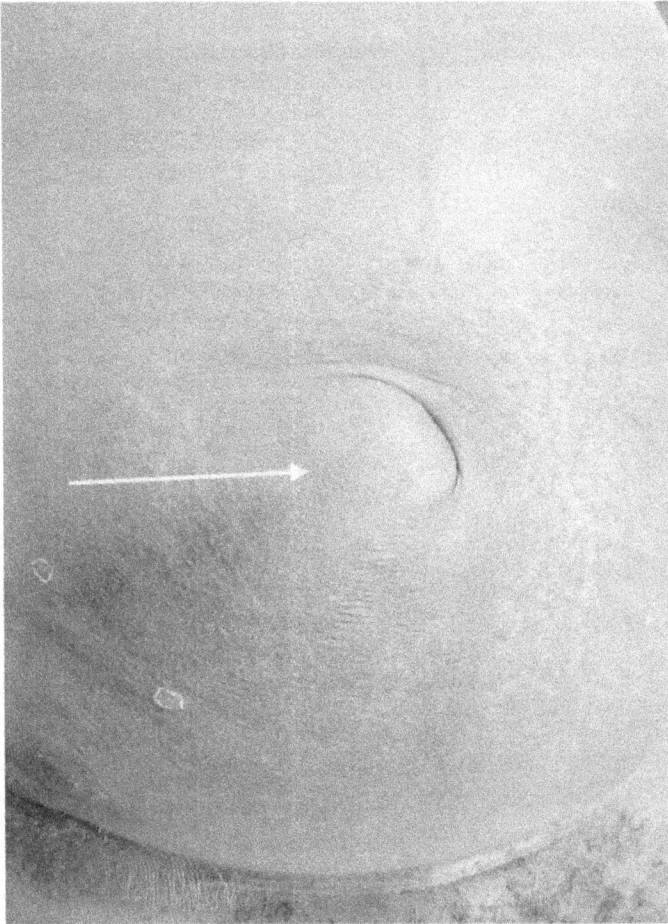

Figure 2.
Non-reducible umbilical tumefaction (image of the Department of Surgery, Gaston Berger University, Saint-Louis, Senegal).

However, the clinical presentation depends mainly on the size of the hernia (neck and sac) and the patient's BMI. In fact, hernias with a small neck or occurring in obese subjects can go unnoticed, especially in an emergency context. In these cases, performing imaging tests is important for an accurate diagnosis.

3.2 Radiological diagnosis

Imaging has an important role in the definitive diagnosis. In fact, clinical examination alone cannot exclude the diagnosis of hernia [11].

Indeed, many hernias are only detectable on imaging (ultrasound or computed tomography) especially when the defect is small or the abdominal fat tissue is important. Besides, imaging can also look for other abdominal wall hernias and more accurately determine the size of the wall defect for an optimization of the treatment.

Imaging also allows to make the differential diagnosis with other, more rare conditions such as abscesses, hematomas or tumors.

Ultrasound is cost effective and efficient. A study has shown that up to 25% of the general population present umbilical hernia when ultrasound is used for diagnosis [12]. This confirms the fact that ultrasound has a much greater sensitivity in detecting umbilical hernias than clinical examination alone. On the other hand, ultrasounds are dependent on the skills of the operator and have a limited contribution when the hernias are large or even with loss of domain. In these cases, the CT scan is of great help. With sagittal and axial reconstructions, CT scan gives more precise information on umbilical hernias (**Figures 3** and **4**).

More recently, some studies have shown that MRI has the best sensitivity and specificity of 92% and 95%, respectively, in the definitive diagnosis of abdominal wall hernias. Indeed, CT and ultrasound cannot completely rule out the presence of a hernia [14]. However, the main drawback of MRI remains the cost-effectiveness and its unavailability in resource limited context.

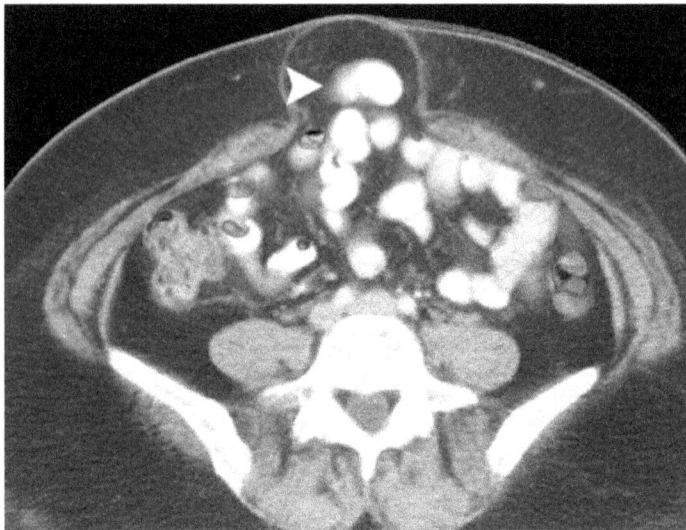

Figure 3.
Axial contrast-enhanced reformatted CT image of an uncomplicated umbilical hernia with small bowel as contents (arrowhead) during Valsalva maneuver [13].

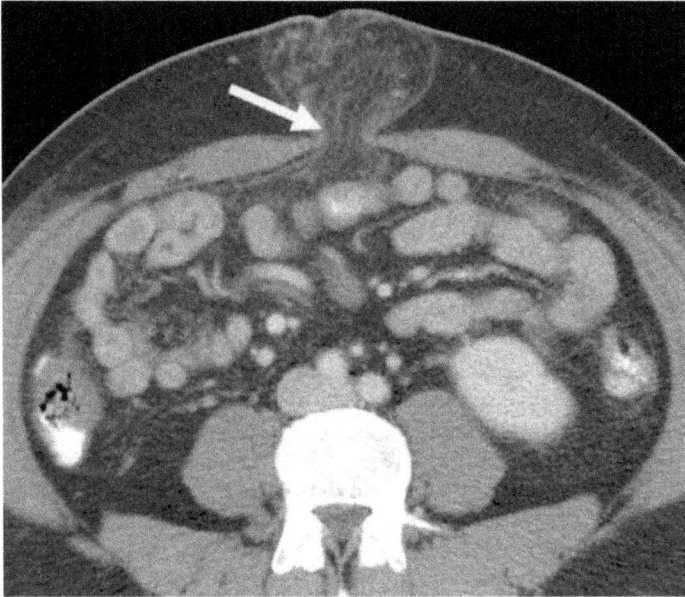

Figure 4.
Axial contrast-enhanced reformatted CT image of an incarcerated umbilical hernia with omental fat as contents (arrow) [13].

4. Treatment

4.1 Preparation of surgery

The treatment of umbilical hernia in adult is surgical. The preparation of the patient is very useful to decrease complications after elective umbilical hernia surgery. In fact, it is recommended smoking cessation for 4–6 weeks and weight loss to a BMI below 35 kg/m2 before surgery [15]. In fact, controlling these factors can reduce the rate of post-operative complications and improve the recovery.

4.2 Anesthesia

All types of anesthesia are possible in umbilical hernia surgery (local, spinal or general anesthesia).

Local anesthesia is feasible in selected patients. Its main advantages lie in the reduction of complications associated with general anesthesia, the reduction of the length of hospital stay (ambulatory surgery) and its cost effectiveness [16, 17]. However, in large hernias or in obese subjects, its use can be difficult.

Rachi-anesthesia is also feasible but often requires a high block which is often incomplete [2].

Thus, general anesthesia is preferred because it allows surgery under better conditions. However, the best technique should be the one based on shared decision-making [15].

4.3 Non operative management

Recently, in developed countries there is an increased interest in "watchful waiting" due to the small risk of strangulation, less than 1% per year [18]. However, a study comparing watchful waiting to surgery showed that, despite no significant difference in terms of mortality in readmission, 19% of non-operated patients will require surgery in the follow up [19]. Due to the risk of complications (strangulation), a watchful waiting approach is not recommended in umbilical hernia and this approach cannot be generalized and depends on the context of care. There is a lack of evidence on the safety of this approach, especially since an adequate follow up is not always possible in resource limited context. Even if watchful waiting is chosen, only asymptomatic umbilical hernia with no esthetic compromise should be non-operatively treated [15].

4.4 Open approach

Open approach is realized with different surgical techniques.

These surgical techniques depend mainly on the use or not of prosthetic material (suture repair or mesh repair).

The suture repairs most performed are simple primary closure and the technique of overlapping the fascia. This second technique was first described by William Mayo and was commonly used [8]. It consists of a plasty of the abdominal wall fascia in "vest-over-pants" (Paletot). However, with a high incidence of recurrence, this approach is less used now.

According to the Guidelines from the European Hernia Society and Americas Hernia Society, it is strongly recommended to use a mesh. In fact, it significantly decreases the rate of recurrence [15]. A randomized clinical trial showed that this rate can be reduced to 1% when mesh is used when compared to suture repair (11%) [20].

Mesh repair is now considered the "gold standard" for umbilical hernia in adults with no associated morbidity factors [21, 22]. In a selected group of patients, suture repair can be performed if the umbilical hernia defect is less than 1 cm.

4.5 Laparoscopic approach

The laparoscopic approach makes it possible to reduce esthetic damage by maintaining the appearance of the umbilicus and avoiding extensive dissections.

In addition, laparoscopy can diagnose other missed hernia during pre-operative procedures, evaluating all of the abdominal wall. Another advantage is the precise evaluation of the umbilical defect in order to use a mesh with the adequate size and overlap of the borders of the defect [23].

The technique consists in the placement of a mesh with a sufficient overlap (3 cm). The recommended site of the mesh placement is pre peritoneal or retro muscular due to the risk of adhesion with intra peritoneal mesh [15].

The prior primary closure of the umbilical defect is not mandatory but its realization may reduce the recurrence rate [24].

The most used mesh is polypropylene because it is cost effective and more available than others. However other types of mesh can also be used (light weight macroporous, composite or dual sides) [8].

Laparoscopic surgery is mainly suggested if the umbilical hernia is large (over 4 cm) [15]. This can decrease the risk of wound infections, post-operative pain, length of hospital stay, and other complications, mostly in patients at risk (obesity, smoking).

4.6 Robotic approach

The use of robotic surgery can improve the results of conventional laparoscopy. Indeed, it allows additional degrees of movement, 3D visualization and better ergonomics for the surgeon. Besides, the attachment of the prosthesis to the anterior abdominal wall, which can be tedious in laparoscopy, is made even easier with the robotic approach [25]. However, longer learning curve, prolonged operative time and cost may be the main limitations of its use.

Hence, in low resource settings, open mesh repair is more feasible. This explains why "tailored surgery" should be the best approach according to the type of patient, the type of hernia, and the context of practice [26].

4.7 Approach in strangulation

The additional morbidity and mortality in emergency surgery require elective surgery whenever it is possible [27]. Evaluation of the contents is mandatory to assess its viability. When there is only ischemia and recoloration after reduction, a simple reduction and parietal repair are done (**Figure 5**). Bowel resection is performed when there is necrosis.

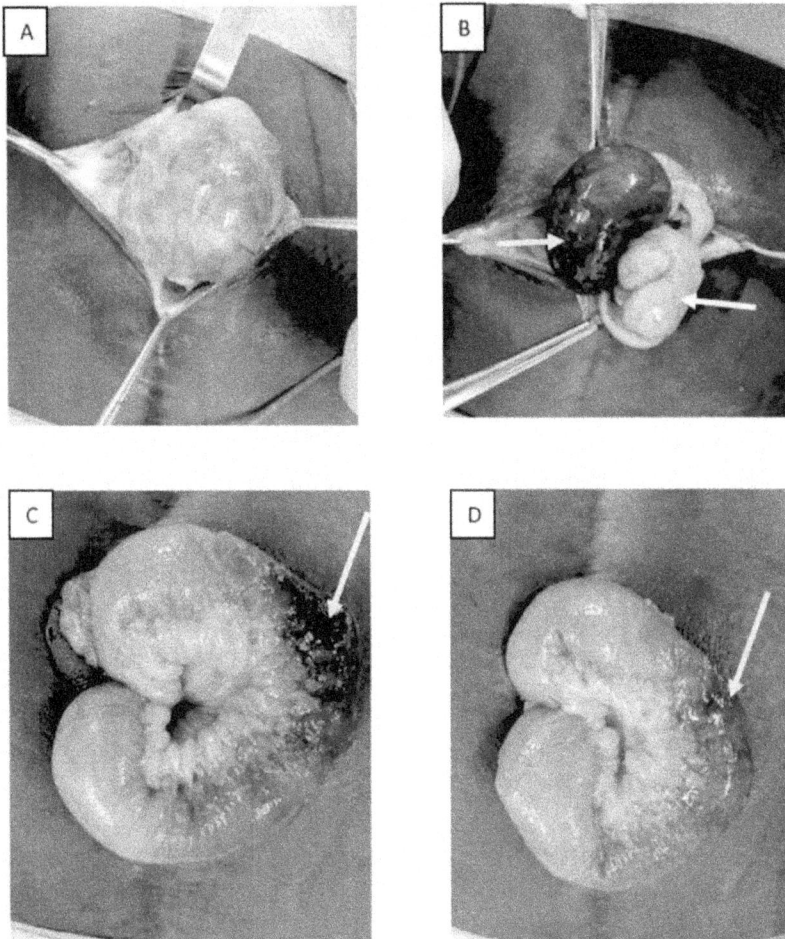

Figure 5.
Per operative image of open approach for a strangulated umbilical hernia: (A) Aspect of the unopened sac; (B) Contents of the hernia with small bowel with ischemia (yellow arrow) and omental fat (white arrow); (C) and (D) Resolution of the small bowel ischemia with recoloration (yellow arrows) (images of the Department of Surgery, Gaston Berger University, Saint-Louis, Senegal).

Both open or laparoscopic approaches are feasible but the open approach is recommended due to the possible necessity of bowel resection and the relative contra-indication of mesh use.

Considering the World Society of Emergency Surgery (WSES) guidelines, the use of mesh will depend on the contamination of the surgical field according to the Centers for Disease Control (CDC) classification. For clean (Class I) or clean-contaminated (Class II) procedures, a mesh can be used. However, for contaminated or infected wounds (Class III and Class IV), suture repair is preferred [28].

4.8 Complications

The most common post-operative complications regardless of the surgical technique are recurrence, superficial surgical site infection and chronic pain or discomfort [29].

Recurrence rate is now low (less than 1%) since the widespread use of mesh. However, mesh related complications are possible and not infrequent (seroma, adhesion, infection, migration or rejection). The removal of the mesh, if possible, should always be considered when mesh related complications occur.

The frequency of these complications is mainly related to co-morbidities, the kind of mesh, the surgical technique and the strategy used to prevent infections [30]. Hence, these complications can be prevented by patient optimization. In fact, obesity, excessive weight and smoking are the mains risk factor for the occurrence of complications [31]. Controlling these factors help reduce the rate of complications.

5. Conclusion

Umbilical hernia remains a relatively common disease in adults. Its diagnosis is clinical and imaging can be used for small defects or in patients with excessive weight. Mesh repair should be preferred for uncomplicated hernia with a defect of more than 1 cm.

Minimally invasive surgery (laparoscopy and robotic) presents important advantages in terms of cosmetic outcome, wound infections, post-operative pain and length of hospital stay.

According to the emergency, the patient characteristics, or the context, "tailored and optimized surgery" should always be used to have the best short and long terms outcomes.

Conflict of interest

"The authors declare no conflict of interest."

Author details

Ibrahima Konaté*, Abdourahmane Ndong and Jacques N. Tendeng
Department of Surgery, Gaston Berger University, Saint Louis, Senegal

*Address all correspondence to: ibrahima.konate@ugb.edu.sn

IntechOpen

References

[1] Coste AH, Jaafar S, Misra S, Parmely JD. Umbilical hernia. InStatPearls [Internet] 2019 Sep 29. StatPearls Publishing.

[2] Velasco M, Garcia-Urena MA, Hidalgo M, Vega V, Carnero FJ. Current concepts on adult umbilical hernia. Hernia. 1999;3(4):233-239.

[3] Kingsnorth A, LeBlanc K. Hernias: inguinal and incisional. Lancet Lond Engl. 2003;362(9395):1561-71.

[4] Al-Salem AH. Abdominal Wall Hernias and Hydroceles. In Atlas of Pediatric Surgery 2020 (pp. 79-98). Springer, Cham.

[5] Ngom G. Umbilical hernia in African children: Same attitude than that of inguinal hernia. J Indian Assoc Pediatr Surg. 2006;11(4):255.

[6] Shankar DA, Itani KMF, O'Brien WJ, Sanchez VM. Factors Associated With Long-term Outcomes of Umbilical Hernia Repair. JAMA Surg. 2017;152(5):461-6.

[7] Dabbas N, Adams K, Pearson K, Royle GT. Frequency of abdominal wall hernias: is classical teaching out of date?. JRSM short reports. 2011 ;2(1):1-6.

[8] Kulaçoğlu H. Current options in umbilical hernia repair in adult patients. Ulus Cerrahi Derg. 2015;31(3):157-61.

[9] Muysoms FE, Miserez M, Berrevoet F, Campanelli G, Champault GG, Chelala E, et al. Classification of primary and incisional abdominal wall hernias. Hernia.2009;13(4):407-14.

[10] Parker SG, Halligan S, Blackburn S, Plumb AAO, Archer L, Mallett S, et al. What Exactly is Meant by "Loss of Domain" for Ventral Hernia? Systematic Review of Definitions. World J Surg. 2019;43(2):396-404.

[11] Bedewi MA, El-sharkawy M. Imaging of Hernias. Hernia. 2017;30:31.

[12] Bedewi MA, El-Sharkawy MS, Al Boukai AA, Al-Nakshabandi N. Prevalence of adult paraumbilical hernia. Assessment by high-resolution sonography: a hospital-based study. Hernia J Hernias Abdom Wall Surg. 2012;16(1):59-62.

[13] Aguirre DA, Santosa AC, Casola G, Sirlin CB. Abdominal Wall Hernias: Imaging Features, Complications, and Diagnostic Pitfalls at Multi–Detector Row CT. RadioGraphics. 2005;25(6):1501-20.

[14] Miller J, Cho J, Michael MJ, Saouaf R, Towfigh S. Role of Imaging in the Diagnosis of Occult Hernias. JAMA Surg. 2014;149(10):1077.

[15] Henriksen NA, Montgomery A, Kaufmann R, Berrevoet F, East B, Fischer J, et al. Guidelines for treatment of umbilical and epigastric hernias from the European Hernia Society and Americas Hernia Society. BJS Br J Surg. 2020;107(3):171-90.

[16] Jairam AP, Kaufmann R, Muysoms F, Jeekel J, Lange JF. The feasibility of local anesthesia for the surgical treatment of umbilical hernia: a systematic review of the literature. Hernia. 2017;21(2):223-231.

[17] Menon VS, Brown TH. Umbilical hernia in adults: day case local anaesthetic repair. J Postgrad Med. 2003;49(2):132.

[18] Leubner KD, Chop WM, Ewigman B, Loven B. What is the risk of bowel strangulation in an adult with an untreated inguinal hernia?. Clinical Inquiries, 2007 (MU). 2007.

[19] Kokotovic D, Sjølander H, Gögenur I, Helgstrand F. Watchful

waiting as a treatment strategy for patients with a ventral hernia appears to be safe. Hernia J Hernias Abdom Wall Surg. 2016;20(2):281-7.

[20] Arroyo A, Garcia P, Perez F, Andreu J, Candela F, Calpena R. Randomized clinical trial comparing suture and mesh repair of umbilical hernia in adults. Br J Surg. 2001;88(10):1321-1323.

[21] Sebastian AA, Perez F, Serrano P, Costa D, Oliver I, Ferrer R, et al. Is prosthetic umbilical hernia repair bound to replace primary herniorrhaphy in the adult patient? Hernia. 2002;6(4):175-177.

[22] Kaufmann R, Halm JA, Eker HH, Klitsie PJ, Nieuwenhuizen J, van Geldere D, et al. Mesh versus suture repair of umbilical hernia in adults: a randomised, double-blind, controlled, multicentre trial. The Lancet. 2018;391(10123):860-869.

[23] Lau H, Patil NG. Umbilical hernia in adults. Surg Endosc Interv Tech. 2003;17(12):2016-2020.

[24] Gonzalez AM, Romero RJ, Seetharamaiah R, Gallas M, Lamoureux J, Rabaza JR. Laparoscopic ventral hernia repair with primary closure versus no primary closure of the defect: potential benefits of the robotic technology. Int J Med Robot. 2015;11(2):120-5.

[25] Chen YJ, Huynh D, Nguyen S, Chin E, Divino C, Zhang L. Outcomes of robot-assisted versus laparoscopic repair of small-sized ventral hernias. Surg Endosc.2017;31(3):1275-9.

[26] Guttadauro A. Introductory Chapter: State of the Art in Hernia Surgery. InTechniques and Innovation in Hernia Surgery 2020 May 27. IntechOpen.

[27] Rind GH, Soomro AH, Ayoob M, Bhatti ZA, Sohu KM. Presentation and Outcome of Strangulated External Abdominal Hernias. JLUMHS. 2010;9(01):04.

[28] Birindelli A, Sartelli M, Di Saverio S, Coccolini F, Ansaloni L, van Ramshorst GH, et al. 2017 update of the WSES guidelines for emergency repair of complicated abdominal wall hernias. World J Emerg Surg. 2017;12(1):37.

[29] Westen M, Christoffersen MW, Jorgensen LN, Stigaard T, Bisgaard T. Chronic complaints after simple sutured repair for umbilical or epigastric hernias may be related to recurrence. Langenbecks Arch Surg. 2014;399(1):65-9.

[30] Falagas ME, Kasiakou SK. Mesh-related infections after hernia repair surgery. Clin Microbiol Infect. 2005;11(1):3-8.

[31] Venclauskas L, Silanskaite J, Kiudelis M. Umbilical hernia: factors indicative of recurrence. Med Kaunas Lith. 2008;44(11):855-9.

Chapter 5

Abdominal Hernia Pain: Chronification Mechanisms after Hernia Surgery

Roberto Sanisidro Torre

Abstract

Groin pain is the most common cause of surgical intervention. There are 3 parameters that increase the chances of chronic pain. On the one hand, starting the surgery with high intensity pain that has not been previously controlled. On the other, insufficient anesthetic and analgesic control during the surgical procedure. Finally, an inadequate management of acute postoperative pain. The presence of groin pain and its poor control before the intervention predisposes to difficulties during the perioperative process. Thus, the appearance of acute postoperative pain not adequately controlled will prevent its remission in a natural way in the usual period (approximately 1 month) and will cause it to progress in intensity and continuity (from 1 month to 3 months after surgery), transforming into a chronic pain (from 3 months after the intervention). In this process of chronification, in which pain goes from nociceptive to neuropathic, different physiological sensitization mechanisms are involved, both peripheral and central. The chronification of the painful process and, ultimately, the therapeutic approach that we will have to use to try to prevent this process depends to a large extent on these modifications that facilitate the change in the nature of pain.

Keywords: groin pain, acute postsurgical pain, chronic postsurgical pain, sensitization

1. Introduction

1.1 Origin of groin pain

It refers to the discomfort that occurs in the groin area of abdominal wall. The most common causes of groin pain include:

- Pulling on a muscle, tendon, or ligament in the leg

- Hernia

- Hip joint disease or injury

Less common causes include:

- Inflammation of the testicle or epididymis and related structures

- Torsion of the spermatic cord attached to the testicle (testicular torsion)

- Tumor of the testicle

- Kidney stones

- Inflammation of the large and small intestine

- Skin infection

- Swelling of the lymph nodes

- Urinary infection

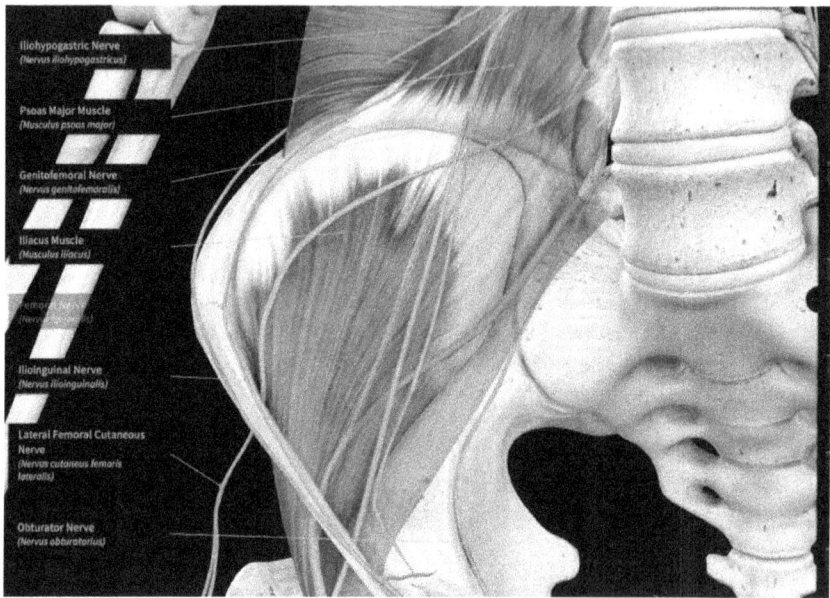

Figure 1.
Nervous system in the groin hernia area (3D 4Medical app).

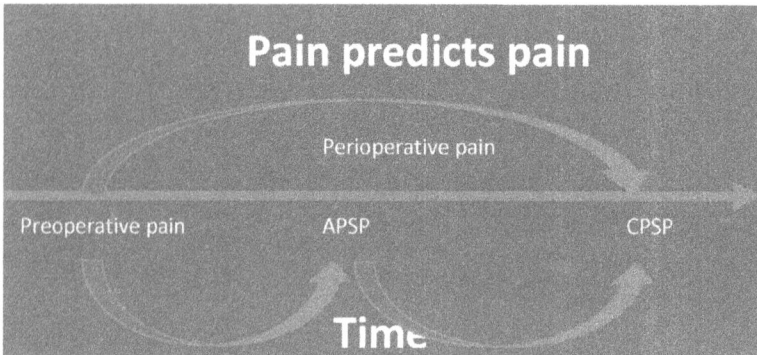

Figure 2.
Predictability of the appearance of CPSP.

This groin pain is perceived, integrated, transmitted and evaluated by neurons and the nervous system, but we have not yet elucidated how this process takes place. Such is the profuse network of nerves that cover the area, that their involvement is a not uncommon phenomenon (**Figure 1**).

In fact, the most frequent surgical reason is inguinal pain resistant to conservative treatments. Besides, poor preoperative pain control is a key factor in developing acute and chronic postsurgical pain (CPSP; **Figure 2**).

2. Risk factors

Each patient who develops CPSP has a specific genotype, medical history, previous experiences, beliefs and psychosocial conditions related to their pain; but, in general, there are some common risk factors in the development of chronic pain.

- *Psychosocial factors*: Anxiety, depression and catastrophizing that surround the patient during the perioperative period.

- *Demographic factors*: In some surgeries, age is a determining factor (i.e. young women for mastectomies [1]). In others, the male gender is more prone than the female [2, 3].

- *Genetic factors*: Several authors point to the relationship of different clinical pathologies such as fibromyalgia, migraine, irritable bowel, irritable bladder, Raynaud's syndrome ... as markers of chronic postsurgical pain [4, 5].

- *Preoperative pain*: The presence of preoperative pain has been correlated in different studies with the development of CPSP. Of all the types of surgical interventions, the hernia procedure stands out for its high preoperative pain rates [6–9].

- *Surgical factors*: Some important surgical factors may be related to the development of CPSP such as:

  ○ Duration of the operation (more than 3 h),

  ○ Surgical technique (laparoscopy vs. open),

  ○ Incision (site and type),

  ○ Experience of the surgeon,

  ○ Center where the intervention is carried out [10].

- *Acute postsurgical pain (APSP)*: Various studies show the importance of optimal APSP control to avoid chronification of postsurgical pain. Among them, surgeries such as groin, breast, hip, knee ... are the most identified [11–13].

However, and despite the fact that there are different studies addressing this issue, the controversy remains dominant. To date, it can only be suggested that they do not play in favor of a better recovery or a lower probability of chronification, in addition to reducing quality of life in the process; but in no case can we establish a universally accepted causal relationship [3, 13–16].

3. Nociception

For the response to a noxious stimulus (be it chemical, thermal, pressure or any other characteristic that can cause pain), there are structures sensitive to those stimuli in the periphery: they are nociceptors [17].

Different classes of afferent nerve fibers are responsible for the communication of nociceptive information and pain:

a. **Type Aβ**: with a myelin sheath, are sensitive fibers responsible for touch and pressure.

b. **Type Aδ**: with a myelin sheath are responsible for the transmission of localized acute pain, temperature and part of the touch.

c. **C fibers**, without myelin sheath are responsible for the transmission of deep diffuse pain, smell, information from some mechanoreceptors, responses of the reflex and postganglionic arcs of the autonomic nervous system.

In a basal state, a noxious stimulus depolarizes a sensory or nociceptor neuron. The stimulation of nociceptors causes the propagation of the nerve stimulus to the dorsal horn of the spinal cord. Control at the spinal level is carried out in the gelatinous substance of Rolando (Rexed plate II) by stimulating inhibitory interneurons (Golgi II type) that cancel or reduce the nociceptive signal towards the lateral spinothalamic tract. In addition, glutamate is released, an excitatory amino acid that binds to a specific receptor, called AMPA and located in a postsynaptic neuron that transmits information to the higher centers of the CNS. Different brain centers are stimulated from the thalamus:

I. *Periaqueductal gray substance (PAGS):* Located in the midbrain, it is one of the most important nuclei and its functions are mediated by the opioid system. Its activation allows the inhibition of the painful process. It is connected with brain structures, with the ascending bundles and sends its projections to structures of the pons such as the nuclei of the raphe magnum.

II. *Nuclei of the raphe magno*: Located in the protuberance, receives connections from the ascending systems and the PAGS. It sends its axons to the first afferent synapse of the posterior horn and its nature is serotonergic.

III. *Cerulean nucleus*: Located on both sides of the fourth ventricle in the bridge. It is noradrenergic in nature.

The prefrontal cortex integrates all the information and the patient feels pain [18]. From these same superior nuclei, descending pathways are set in motion and reach the dorsal horn of the medulla again releasing endogenous inhibitory substances (mainly opioids and GABA). These inhibitory substances act by modulating the transmission of the stimulus: on the one hand, by decreasing the release of glutamate, and on the other, by hyperpolarizing the membrane of the postsynaptic neuron [19]. Inhibitory interneurons also come into play, which by releasing endogenous opioids, mimic and potentiate the inhibitory effect of the descending pathways.

3.1 Nociceptive pain

Refers to pain that is associated with actual or threatened damage to non-neural tissue and involves the activation of peripheral nociceptors (IASP Taxonomy, 2015). There are three major forms of nociceptive pain:

3.1.1 Somatic

Includes all pain originating from non-visceral structures, (i.e. skull, meninges, and teeth) and is the most common cause of consultation for almost all specialties, especially those dedicated to the locomotor system.

3.1.2 Myofascial

Extremely frequent, although in many cases it is not diagnosed as such. It is a neuromuscular dysfunction with a tendency to chronicity. It consists of a regional pain disorder, which affects the muscles and fasciae, so that the muscles involved have trigger points as essential components. In addition, regional and segmental autonomous alterations may coexist.

3.1.3 Visceral

Dull, diffuse and poorly localized pain, referred to an area of the body surface, being frequently accompanied by an intense motor and autonomic (sympathetic) reflex response. The stimuli that can produce visceral pain are: spasm of the smooth muscle (hollow viscera), distension and ischemia.

4. Neuropathy

Sometimes there is no relationship between the painful stimulus and the response that it originates in the CNS: it is then when a very important amplification of the nociceptive signal occurs, and this phenomenon is known as neuronal sensitization or neuropathy, so that the information transmitted to the brain causes a disproportionate pain reaction. This derangement occurs both at the peripheral and central levels.

4.1 Neuropathic pain

Persistent pain becomes a pathological state that includes a series of elements that facilitate its generation and persistence over time. For this reason, any process that injures nerve tissues or causes neuronal dysfunction can produce neuropathic pain (NP). NP is qualitatively characterized by the absence of a causal relationship between injury and pain. Its etiology is very diverse and the relationship between etiology, pathophysiological mechanisms and symptoms is complex. NP differs from nociceptive pain in several aspects (**Table 1**).

The balance between arousal and inhibition of the somatosensory system is dynamic and is influenced by context, behaviors, emotions, expectations, and pathology. In NP this equilibrium is broken and a loss in inhibitory currents has been demonstrated, with dysfunction in the mechanisms of production and release of GABA, a decrease in μ-opioid receptors in the dorsal root ganglia, and less receptivity to opioids in the spinal neurons. In summary, the neuronal pathological

	Nociceptive (somatic / visceral)	Neuropathic
Official definition	Pain caused by activation of peripheral / visceral nociceptors	Pain caused by PNS / CNS dysfunction
Mechanism	Natural physiological transduction (nociceptor)	Ectopic pulse generation
Symptom location	Local pain + referred	Territory of innervation of the affected nerve pathway
	No neurological topography	
Quality of symptoms	Common painful sensations of daily life - easy verbal description (i.e. Head ache, belly ache...)	New, unfamiliar, aberrant sensations: difficult verbal description (i.e. burning, electrical...)
	Normal neurological examination: response and aggression correspond	Hypo / hypersensitivity: response and aggression do not correspond
Treatment	Effective: conventional analgesia	Partially effective: antiepileptics, antidepressants

Adapted from Serra Catafau, Treatise on neuropathic pain (Adapted from SGADOR Handbook).

Table 1.
Differences between nociceptive and neuropathic pain.

process changes in the course of injury and its pathophysiological mechanisms are evolutionary. The mechanisms that trigger NP produce:

- Local inflammation

- Glia cell activation

- Changes in neuronal plasticity of nociceptive pain-transmitting pathways

5. Acute pain

Acute pain is an experience, usually of sudden onset, of short duration in time and with remission parallel to the cause that produces it. There is a close temporal and causal relationship with tissue injury or nociceptive stimulation caused by disease. Its duration ranges from a few minutes to several weeks. Acute pain has been attributed a "protective" function, its presence acts by preventing the individual from developing behaviors that may increase the injury or leads him to adopt those that minimize or reduce its impact. The fundamental emotional response is anxiety, with less involvement of other psychological components. Its characteristics offer important help in establishing the etiological diagnosis and selecting the most appropriate treatment. Its presence follows a classic treatment scheme such as Pain-Symptom. The most common causes of acute pain are:

1. Visceral pain

    i. Gastrointestinal

    ii. Biliary

    iii. Urological

    iv. Cardiovascular

    v. Pulmonary

    vi. Nervous system

    vii. Pancreatic

    viii. Gynecological

2. Muscle Skeletal Pain

    i. Arthropathies

    ii. Chest wall pain

    iii. Fractures

    iv. Costochondritis

    v. Tendinitis

3. Oral pain

4. Burn pain

5. Postoperative pain

6. Chronic pain

Chronic pain extends beyond the tissue injury or organic involvement with which, initially, there was a relationship. It can also be related to the persistence and repetition of episodes of acute pain, with the progression of the disease, with the appearance of complications thereof and with degenerative changes in bone and

	Acute Pain	Chronic pain
Purpose	Initial-biological	Initial-destructive
Duration	Temporary	Persistent
Generator mechanism	Unifactorial	Multifactorial
Affected component	Organic+++Psychic+	Organic+Psychic+++
Organic response	Adrenergic: raise in heart rate, arterial hypertension, sweating, pupillary dilation	Vegetative: anorexy, constipation, less lybid, insomnia
Affective component	Anxiety	Depression
Physical exhaustion	No	Yes
Therapeutic goal	Cure	Relief and adaptation

Table 2.
Differences between acute and chronic pain.

musculoskeletal structures. Examples of this are cancer, secondary pathological fractures, osteoarthritis, postherpetic neuralgia, etc.

Chronic pain does not prevent or avoid damage to the body. Both their nature and their intensity show great variability over time, in many cases the complaints are perceived as disproportionate to the underlying disease. The most frequent repercussions in the psychological sphere involve anxiety, anger, fear, frustration or depression, which, in turn, contribute to further increasing pain perception. The socio-family, labor and economic repercussions are multiple and generate important changes in the lives of the people who suffer from it and their families: disability and dependency. The need to use drugs to relieve pain becomes a potential risk factor for use, abuse and self-prescription, not only of analgesics, but also tranquilizers, antidepressants and other drugs.

In its management, in addition to the physical aspects of pain, the other components, emotional, affective, behavioral and social, must be taken into account. The treatment scheme is complicated, we are facing the Pain-Syndrome (**Table 2**).

7. Postsurgical groin pain

7.1 Acute postsurgical groin pain

All surgical intervention is associated with acute postsurgical pain (APSP) whose intensity decreases during the first days and weeks, in parallel with the tissue repair process. However, sometimes this pain lasts longer than is reasonable in relation to the surgical procedure. This fact can lead to the appearance of severe and disabling chronic pain syndromes, frequently associated with certain surgical procedures.

The definition of chronic postoperative pain (CPSP) does not find a consensus among the different authors in the literature reviewed. The most commonly used definition continues to be that of McRae [20, 21] based on the following aspects:

a. pain with a minimum duration of two months after a surgical procedure

b. after excluding other etiologies of pain

c. ruled out any pre-existing cause of pain (**Figure 3**).

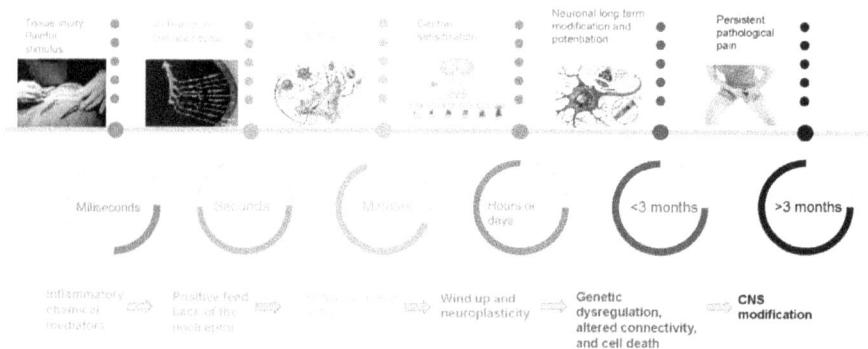

Figure 3.
Temporal evolution of postsurgical pain (adapted from Woolf and salter, science 2000; 288: 1765 [22]).

CPSP originates from the injury to the nerves and tissues inherent in the surgical process. During the immediate postsurgical period appears the breakthrough pain limited to the surgical site and its vicinity and develops through the direct activation of nociceptors, the inflammatory process and, in some cases, of direct nerve injury [23]. For this reason, the patient will present pain in the area of the surgical scar (primary hyperalgesia) and around it (secondary hyperalgesia). These changes are usually reversible and the normal sensitivity of the nociceptive system will then be restored. This type of pain, APSP, has a known beginning and an end in direct relation to tissue repair. In addition, it responds effectively to non-steroidal anti-inflammatory drugs, paracetamol, and minor or major opioids.

In the event of nerve injury during surgery, the neuropathic component of pain can immediately develop and persist in the absence of any noxious peripheral stimuli or ongoing peripheral inflammation [24]. The prerequisite for the development of CPSP is an injury to the major nerves that run through the surgical site. However, in a small group of patients, an ongoing inflammatory response may help maintain inflammatory pain and lead to a CPSP, such as that occurs after inguinal mesh hernia repair [25]. During progression from APSP to CPSP after inguinal hernia surgery:

- 7% of patients present severe acute pain the first 24 h;

- 14% of patients present subacute pain that could last until 8 weeks after surgery;

- 12% of patients present CPSP that could last until 12 months after surgery (80% of whom present Neuropathic component)

The incidence of chronic pain after inguinal hernia surgery rates from 5–63%, with an estimated incidence of severe chronic pain (VAS > 4) between 2% and 4%.

7.2 Inguinal chronic pain

Inguinal hernia surgery can trigger a post-herniorrhaphy chronic inguinal pain syndrome, which can occur in up to 10% of the interventions performed [21].

The symptoms of postherniorrhaphy neuropathic inguinodynia consist of pain, paresthesias, allodynia (sensation of pain in the presence of non-harmful stimuli such as touch or pressure), pain radiating to the scrotal area, labia majora of the vagina and Scarpa's triangle. This symptomatology also worsens with walking or hyperextension of the hip and decreases with decubitus and flexion of the thigh. These last aspects of the symptomatology make us see that the affectation of the nervous tract is the main actor of the chronic pain postherniorrhaphy [26].

There are three types of causes for the appearance of this painful syndrome:

   i. Non-neuropathic

     a. Reaction of the periosteum of the pubis

     b. Keloid scar formation

     c. Direct pressure exerted by bent or wrinkled prosthetic material (mesh) [27].

ii. Neuropathic

    a. Fibrosis of the perineurium of the nerves that run along the inguinal path (ilioinguinal nerve and genital branch of the genitofemoral nerve)

    b. Compression of these by suture material, staples or prosthetic material

iii. *Direct injury to the nervous tract in a complete or incomplete manner.* It can be produced by traction, direct cutting with a scalpel, or excessive thermocoagulation.

7.2.1 Peripheral sensitization

Peripheral sensitization involves lowering the discharge threshold from the peripheral terminal of the nociceptor. The molecules released in response to tissue damage and the activation of cells in the environment such as keratinocytes, mast cells, lymphocytes, platelets or the nociceptor itself, are called inflammatory soup (Substance P, calcitonin gene receptor protein [CGRP], quinines, amines, prostaglandins, growth factors, chemokines, cytokines, ATP, protons, etc.). These molecules induce morphological and functional changes in the neuron, which consequently generate an increase in the expression of structures such as the Na^{2+} channels and transient receptor potential cation channel subfamily V member 1 [TRPV1]; or molecules such as neuropeptides, or brain-derived neurotrophic factor [BDNF]. The interaction of these molecules with the different membrane receptors initiates an activation cascade of intracellular second messengers that modify the firing capacity of the cell, the final consequence being a greater capacity to respond to stimuli. This circumstance translates clinically into the following processes: hyperalgesia, allodynia, and spontaneous pain.

Spontaneous pain can be caused by:

i. An abnormal response to stimuli that normally do not cause harm (arterial heartbeat, increased temperature)

ii. Ectopic discharges from the damaged nociceptor itself

iii. Those produced by surrounding healthy fibers in response to the release of TNFα by damaged Schwann cells

At present, it is proposed a new state of the nociceptor, called "priming", in which, a sensitized nociceptor, after a few hours will have a normal response to physiological stimuli, but will have an increased response to stimuli derived from inflammation. This state lasts for weeks and the hyperalgesic response to inflammatory agents is greater, which could be a possible explanation for the maintenance of chronic pain.

In a situation in which nociceptive information continues to be sent from the periphery to the dorsal horn of the spinal cord, the nociceptive neuron itself sends, from its soma (without the need for external stimulation) substance P and peptide related to the calcitonin gene (PRCG). These substances bind to neutrophils, mast cells and basophils, and release pro-inflammatory molecules: cytosines, bradykinins, histamines, cyclooxygenases, prostaglandins, eicosanoids and nerve growth factor (NGF). All this "inflammatory soup" produces changes in pH, release of ATP from injured cells, synthesis and release of nitric oxide (NO), etc., which induces amplification of the signal towards the spinal cord and higher centers and causes what is known as peripheral sensitization, which contributes in a very important manner to the maintenance of chronic pain.

7.2.2 Central sensitization

If the nociceptive impulses are of great intensity or are sustained over time, plastic changes occur in the neurons of the posterior horn that facilitate the transmission of the nociceptive impulse. These changes in functionality are called central sensitization and cause specific clinical manifestations. It may represent the anatomical and physiological substrate to the fact of persistence of pain in the absence of peripheral nociceptive impulses in chronic pain, since the state of hyper-reactivity of the system would allow to explain the autonomous activity of the system in the absence of peripheral stimulus. In general terms, the following changes can be considered, which can all occur simultaneously or simply manifest some of them:

I. Disinhibition of the N-methyl-D-aspartate (NMDA) receptor by release of the Mg^{2+} ion at the first medullary synapse

II. Access of peripheral Aβ fibers to the nociceptive system. It is one of the causes of the phenomenon of allodynia

III. Dysregulation of the GABAergic system of inhibitory interneurons, which finally produces an alteration in the current of the Cl^- channel.

IV. Activation of the glia with the release of pro-analgesic substances

V. Alteration of the regulatory capacity of the downstream system

There is also the release of glutamate, which binds to specific receptors, which are not expressed in situations of acute pain. When activated, they contribute not only to depolarize the postsynaptic neuron, but also to generate a series of intracellular changes, which will increase the nociceptive signal. In response to peripheral sensitization, the primary afferent pathways also release substance P, resulting in an increase in signal. In situations of chronic pain there is also a reorganization of the neuronal structure: axonal collateral branches appear that increase the amount of nociceptive afferent signal.

On the other hand, a loss of efficacy of the inhibition produced by the descending pathways has been described, with a decrease in the release of endogenous opioids, and even cellular degeneration of those descending neurons, which indirectly also increases the nociceptive signal that is send to higher centers.

All these changes greatly amplify and sustain the nociceptive signal produced in the dorsal horn of the spinal cord, producing what is known as central sensitization.

The main clinical manifestations of nervous sensitization are hyperalgesia and allodynia phenomena, with the consequent increase in the extension of the painful area.

The presence of sensitization leads to the appearance of vicious circles in which there is a continuous sending of the afferent signal from the periphery to the brain centers in the absence of stimuli that generate them. This sustained stimulation leads to adaptive changes in the brain, such that the brain remains active even in the absence of noxious peripheral stimulus.

This continuous brain overexcitation conditions the effectiveness of the integrative pain response of the higher centers and the inhibitory descending pathway, in such a way that there is no inhibition proportional to the ascending amplified stimulus and the pain becomes chronic. This "centralizing" effect of the neuronal sensitization of nociceptors is one of the most relevant chronifying factors in the postoperative period of surgeries that present moderate to severe acute pain, that is not adequately controlled.

7.2.3 Pharmacological strategies

The type of pain, its location, duration and intensity determine the pharmacological approach (**Figure 4**).

- **Drugs that target peripheral sensitization**: such as topical **capsaicin** (i.e. 8% capsaicin patch); topical lidocaine (i.e. 5% lidocaine patch); NSAIDs; paracetamol and local anesthetics.

- **Drugs that target central sensitization:** such as serotonin reuptake inhibitors (SSRIs); tapentadol; tramadol; opioids; calcium channel ligands; adjuvants; tricyclic antidepressants; anticonvulsants and COX-2.

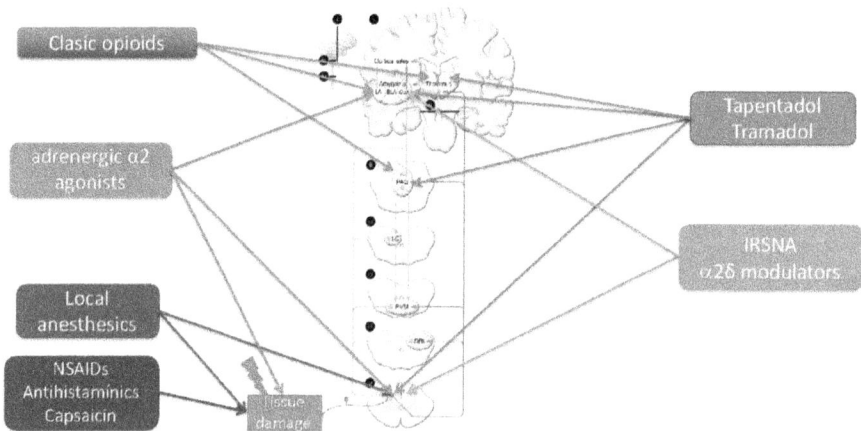

Figure 4.
Pharmacological approach to chronic pain.

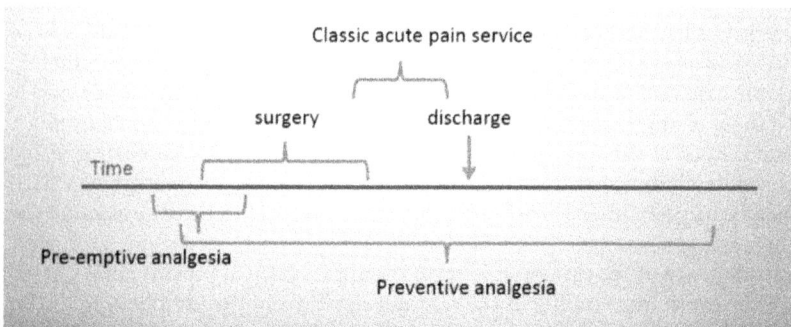

Figure 5.
Perioperative analgesia.

7.2.4 Preventive strategies

Blocking the pain signal before it reaches the central nervous system prior to surgery will prevent the development of central sensitization. The times that include the first consultation, the referral to the specialist, the decision of surgical treatment, the pre-anesthetic consultation and the appointment for surgery would favor peripheral and central sensitization if pain is not controlled, making the pain chronic and making it independent of the injury.

7.2.5 Rescue strategies

Using aggressive perioperative analgesia (antihyperalgesics, regional blocks, and multimodal analgesia) during the peri-surgical period could reduce the incidence of CPSP (**Figure 5**).

7.2.6 Are all the operations necessary or appropriate?

Chronic pain is common after hernia surgery. Patients with pain before the operation benefit from surgery, but some patients who have no pain before hernia repair surgery develop significant groin pain later. Watchful waiting has proven to be safe [28] and profitable [29] in patients with asymptomatic inguinal hernia. It is a theme of debate whether surgery is appropriate in asymptomatic hernias and possibly in some other interventions as well.

8. Summary

CPSP is a common entity in interventional procedures today. Progress continues in the standardization of prevention and treatment strategies for this delicate problem in the technical and organizational sphere.

The improvement efforts aim to:

- Early identification of patients with preoperative pain who need intervention.

- Avoid delaying this intervention as far as possible, and if there is a delay, provide adequate pain management until the time of surgery.

- At the time of the intervention, determine the least invasive and most appropriate surgical technique for the pathology.

- Implement the most appropriate perioperative anesthetic and analgesic techniques for the patient.

- Once intervened, individualize postoperative analgesia so that APSP is as low as possible, thus avoiding, as far as possible, chronic pain.

Acknowledgements

Thanks to Merche and Eduardo, for giving me the opportunity to study without worrying about anything else. To Monica, for her patience in preparing this chapter and to Alaitz and Inhar, for their fun distractions.

Conflict of interest

I declare that I have no conflict of interests.

Author details

Roberto Sanisidro Torre
Experimental Surgery Department, UPV/EHU, Bilbao, Spain

*Address all correspondence to: roberto.sanisidro@gmail.com

IntechOpen

References

[1] Tasmuth T, von Smitten K, Hietanen P, Kataja M, Kalso E. Pain and other symptoms after different treatment modalities of breast cancer. Ann Oncol. 1995;6:453-459.

[2] Caumo W, Schmidt AP, Schneider CN, Bergmann J, Iwamoto CW, Adamatti LC, et al. Preoperative predictors of moderate to intense acute postoperative pain in patients undergoing abdominal surgery. Acta Anaesthesiol Scand. 2002;46:1265-71.

[3] Katz J, Poleshuck EL, Andrus CH, Hogan LA, Jung BF, Kulick DI, et al. Risk factors for acute pain and its persistence following breast cancer surgery. Pain. 2005;119:16-25.

[4] Courtney CA, Duffy K, Serpell MG, O'Dwyer PJ. Outcome of patients with severe chronic pain following repair of groin hernia. Br J Surg. 2002;89:1310-4.

[5] Wright D, Paterson C, Scott N, Hair A, O'Dwyer PJ. Five-year follow-up of patients undergoing laparoscopic or open groin hernia repair: a randomized controlled trial. Ann Surg. 2002;235:333-7.

[6] Liem MS, van Duyn EB, van der Graaf Y, van Vroonhoven TJ. Recurrences after conventional anterior and laparoscopic inguinal hernia repair: a randomized comparison. Ann Surg. 2003;237:136-41.

[7] Poobalan AS, Bruce J, King PM, Chambers WA, Krukowski ZH, Smith WC. Chronic pain and quality of life following open inguinal hernia repair. Br J Surg. 2001;88:1122-6.

[8] Wright D, Paterson C, Scott N, Hair A, O'Dwyer PJ. Five-year follow-up of patients undergoing laparoscopic or open groin hernia repair: a

randomized controlled trial. Ann Surg. 2002;235:333-7.

[9] Page B, Paterson C, Young D, O'Dwyer PJ. Pain from primary inguinal hernia and the effect of repair on pain. Br J Surg. 2002;89:1315-8.

[10] Peters ML, Sommer M, de Rijke JM, Kessels F, Heineman E, Patijn J, et al. Somatic and psychologic predictors of longterm unfavorable outcome after surgical intervention. Ann Surg. 2007;245: 487-94.

[11] Aasvang E, Kehlet H. Chronic postoperative pain: the case of inguinal herniorrhaphy. Br J Anaesth. 2005;95:69-76.

[12] Poleshuck EL, Katz J, Andrus CH, Hogan LA, Jung BF, Kulick DI, et al. Risk factors for chronic pain following breast cancer surgery: a prospective study. J Pain. 2006;7:626-34.

[13] Nikolajsen L, Brandsborg B, Lucht U, Jensen TS, Kehlet H. Chronic pain following total hip arthroplasty: a nationwide questionnaire study. Acta Anaesthesiol Scand. 2006;50:495-500.

[14] Tasmuth T, Estlanderb AM, Kalso E. Effect of present pain and mood on the memory of past postoperative pain in women treated surgically for breast cancer. Pain. 1996;68:343-7.

[15] Hanley MA, Jensen MP, Ehde DM, Hoffman AJ, Patterson DR, Robinson LR. Psychosocial predictors of long-term adjustment to lower-limb amputation and phantom limb pain. Disabil Rehabil. 2004;26:882-93.

[16] Poobalan AS, Bruce J, Smith WC, King PM, Krukowski ZH, Chambers WA. A review of chronic pain after inguinal herniorrhaphy. Clin J Pain. 2003;19:48-54.

[17] Julius D, Basbaum AI. Molecular mechanisms of nociception. Nature 2001; 413:203-10.

[18] Doubell TP, Mannion RJ, Woolf CJ. The dorsal Horn: state-dependent sensory processing, plasticity and the generation of pain. En: Wall P, Melzack R, editors. Textbook of Pain. 4th ed. Philadelphia: Churcill Livingstone; 2003. p. 165-82.

[19] Mason P. Deconstructing endogenous pain modulation. J Neurophysiol 2005; 94:1659-63.

[20] Macrae WA.Davies HTO. Chronic postsurgical pain. Epidemiology of pain. Seattle: IASP Press 1999. p.125-42.

[21] Macrae WA. Chronic pain after surgery. Br J Anaesth 2001;87:88-98.

[22] Woolf CJ, Salter M. Neuronal plasticity: increasing the gain in pain. Science 2000; 288: 1765-9.

[23] Kehlet H, Jensen TS, Woolf CJ. Persistent postsurgical pain: risk factors andprevention. Lancet 2006; 367:1618-25.

[24] Jung BF, Ahrendt GM, Oaklander AL, DworkinRH. Neuropathic pain following breast cancer surgery: proposed classification and research update. Pain 2003; 104:1-13.

[25] Aasvang E, Kehlet H. Chronic postoperative pain: the case of inguinal herniorrhaphy. Br J Anaesth 2005; 95:69-76.

[26] Amid PK. Causes, prevention, and surgical treatment of postherniorrhaphy neuropathic inguinodynia: triple neurectomy with proximal end implantation. Hernia 2004 Dec;8(4):343-9.

[27] Amid PK. The Lichtenstein repair in 2002: an overview of causes of recurrence after Lichtenstein tension-free hernioplasty. Hernia 2003;7:101-15.

[28] Poobalan AS, Bruce J, Smith WC, King PM, Krukowski ZH, Chambers WA. A review of chronic pain after inguinal herniorrhaphy. Clin J Pain. 2003;19:48-54.

[29] Stroupe KT, Manheim LM, Luo P, Giobbie-Hurder A, Hynes DM, Jonasson O, et al. Tension-free repair versus watchful waiting for men with asymptomatic or minimally symptomatic inguinal hernias: a cost-effectiveness analysis. J Am Coll Surg. 2006;203:458-68.